Quit Smoking

How to Stop Your Smoking Addiction

(Your Cigarette Addiction the Easy Way without Painful Nicotine Withdrawal)

Victor Bergeron

Published By **Jenna Olsen**

Victor Bergeron

All Rights Reserved

Quit Smoking: How to Stop Your Smoking Addiction (Your Cigarette Addiction the Easy Way without Painful Nicotine Withdrawal)

ISBN 978-1-7382957-4-6

No part of this guidebook shall be reproduced in any form without permission in writing from the publisher except in the case of brief quotations embodied in critical articles or reviews.

Legal & Disclaimer

The information contained in this book is not designed to replace or take the place of any form of medicine or professional medical advice. The information in this book has been provided for educational & entertainment purposes only.

The information contained in this book has been compiled from sources deemed reliable, and it is accurate to the best of the Author's knowledge; however, the Author cannot guarantee its accuracy and validity and cannot be held liable for any errors or omissions. Changes are periodically made to this book. You must consult your doctor or get professional medical advice before using any of the suggested remedies, techniques, or information in this book.

Upon using the information contained in this book, you agree to hold harmless the Author from and against any damages, costs, and expenses, including any legal fees potentially resulting from the application of any of the information provided by this guide. This disclaimer applies to any damages or injury caused by the use and application, whether directly or indirectly, of any advice or information presented, whether for breach of contract, tort, negligence, personal injury, criminal intent, or under any other cause of action.

You agree to accept all risks of using the information presented inside this book. You need to consult a professional medical practitioner in order to ensure you are both able and healthy enough to participate in this program.

Table Of Contents

Chapter 1: Understanding Addiction 1

Chapter 2: Building A Support System 13

Chapter 3: Creating A Quit Plan 21

Chapter 4: Healthy Habits 33

Chapter 5: Dealing With Cravings 48

Chapter 6: Overcoming Challenges 59

Chapter 7: Celebrating Milestones 63

Chapter 8: Motivational Anecdotes 73

Chapter 9: Understanding Smoking Addiction 77

Chapter 10: Setting Personal Goals 85

Chapter 11: Identifying And Managing Cravings 95

Chapter 12: Behavioral Changes For Smoking Cessation 107

Chapter 13: Dealing With Relapses 121

Chapter 14: The Disconcerting Beginning 133

Chapter 15: Neuroscience Of Tobacco..149

Chapter 16: The Butterfly Effect 162

Chapter 17: Controlling Addiction From
The Micro Biota......................................176

Chapter 1: Understanding Addiction

Nicotine addiction is a complex device stimulated thru each natural and mental factor. Understanding the technological records at the back of nicotine addiction can shed moderate on why quitting may be tough for lots individuals. Here's a breakdown of the vital thing components:

Nicotine and the Brain:

When a person smokes, nicotine is unexpectedly absorbed into the bloodstream via the lungs and reaches the thoughts inside seconds.

In the brain, nicotine binds to specific receptors, greater often than not in the praise middle known as the nucleus accumbens.

The binding of nicotine to the ones receptors triggers the discharge of neurotransmitters, inclusive of dopamine, that is related to pleasure and praise.

Dopamine Release:

Dopamine is a neurotransmitter that performs a essential function in reinforcing behaviors associated with pride and reward.

Nicotine stimulates the discharge of dopamine within the mind, growing a experience of delight and satisfaction.

Reward Pathway Activation:

With repeated exposure to nicotine, the mind adapts with the aid of the usage of adjusting the sensitivity of its reward pathways.

Over time, the mind turns into reliant on nicotine to hold a fantastic degree of pride, foremost to the development of dependence.

Tolerance and Dependence:

As the thoughts adapts to the regular presence of nicotine, individuals also can broaden tolerance, requiring extra nicotine to gain the equal quality effects.

Dependence takes area at the same time as the thoughts is based on nicotine to function typically, and the absence of nicotine results in withdrawal signs and symptoms and signs.

Withdrawal Symptoms:

When a person tries to surrender smoking, they'll experience withdrawal signs and signs and symptoms due to the fact the mind adjusts to the absence of nicotine.

Common withdrawal symptoms and signs embody irritability, cravings, problem concentrating, prolonged urge for food, and temper swings.

Cravings and Triggers:

Nicotine addiction is often associated with environmental and situational triggers, at the side of strain, social situations, or specific sports activities related to smoking.

Exposure to the ones triggers can evoke robust cravings, making it hard for humans to cease.

Long-Term Changes in the Brain:

Prolonged nicotine use can bring about structural and useful changes in the thoughts, affecting areas answerable for selection-making, impulse manipulate, and judgment.

Understanding the technological expertise in the back of nicotine addiction underscores the significance of complete strategies for quitting. Behavioral interventions, counseling, resource businesses, and pharmacological aids like nicotine replacement remedy (NRT) can help individuals deal with each the bodily and mental components of dependancy, improving their opportunities of correctly quitting smoking.

The mental components of smoking play a sizeable position in the development and protection of dependancy. These factors embody the emotional, social, and cognitive elements that contribute to smoking behavior. Understanding the ones intellectual elements is crucial for individuals seeking to surrender smoking. Here are a few key highbrow components of smoking:

Stress and Coping Mechanisms:

Many people flip to smoking as a manner to cope with strain. Nicotine, a stimulant in tobacco, can brief alleviate stress and tension.

Smoking becomes associated with stress alleviation, developing a mental dependence on cigarettes as a coping mechanism.

Habitual Behavior:

Smoking often becomes ingrained in each day physical activities and behavior. For example, humans also can accomplice smoking with particular sports activities like having a cup of coffee, taking a destroy, or socializing.

Breaking the ones regular establishments is a vital element of quitting smoking.

Social and Environmental Influences:

Smoking is often a social interest, and those may additionally furthermore smoke in reaction to social cues or peer pressure.

Being in environments in which smoking is not unusual can trigger the choice to smoke, emphasizing the want to cope with social and environmental elements for the duration of the quitting way.

Emotional Associations:

Smoking can come to be connected to numerous feelings, which include joy, sadness, boredom, or birthday celebration. The act of smoking may be used to decorate extraordinary emotions or alleviate horrific ones.

Identifying and locating opportunity strategies to manipulate emotions is a key element of overcoming intellectual dependence on smoking.

Self-Identity and Smoking:

For a few human beings, smoking will become intertwined with their self-identification. The perception that smoking defines them or makes them extra confident can be a barrier to quitting.

Shifting one's self-notion and building a cutting-edge, smoke-unfastened identification is crucial inside the intellectual aspect of quitting.

Fear of Weight Gain:

Some human beings fear weight advantage after quitting smoking, as nicotine can suppress urge for food and growth metabolism.

Addressing worries about weight advantage and adopting wholesome manner of existence conduct are important in overcoming this psychological barrier.

Perceived Benefits of Smoking:

Smokers regularly recognize blessings in smoking, which include improved attention, relaxation, or extra suitable social interactions.

Challenging the ones perceptions and finding alternative, extra healthy strategies to gain those blessings is crucial within the quitting method.

Mindfulness and Awareness:

Developing mindfulness and being aware about the motivations and triggers for smoking can empower humans to make aware picks and withstand the urge to smoke.

Addressing the mental factors of smoking consists of not only breaking the bodily addiction to nicotine but additionally reprogramming the associated behaviors, thoughts, and emotions. Behavioral treatment alternatives, counseling, and help organizations can be effective in assisting human beings navigate and triumph over those psychological worrying situations on the journey to end smoking.

Setting Your Quit Date

Choosing a big stop smoking date may be an critical step for your adventure to become smoke-loose. Here are some tips that will help you choose a date that holds private importance and complements your opportunities of achievement:

Personal Milestones:

Consider tying your quit date to a big non-public milestone, which encompass a birthday, anniversary, or unique occasion. Associating your surrender date with immoderate excellent activities can upload motivation and make the date greater memorable.

Health Awareness Days:

Select a prevent date that aligns with a health-related observance, just like the Great American Smokeout (0.33 Thursday in November) or World No Tobacco Day (May 31st). Participating in these sports can provide a feel of community guide and worldwide reputation.

Financial Milestones:

Calculate how a first rate deal cash you spend on cigarettes every day and set your prevent date to coincide with a financial milestone, similar to the start of a current month or pay period. This can encourage you with the useful useful resource of highlighting the monetary benefits of quitting.

Seasonal Changes:

Some people discover it beneficial to give up smoking in the path of a exchange of season, collectively with the begin of spring or fall. The smooth begin related to seasonal changes can feature a symbolic instance of your commitment to a greater fit way of life.

Personal Significance:

Choose a date that has non-public because of this for you. It might be the anniversary of a significant life occasion, the day you commenced smoking (to reclaim manage), or any date that resonates collectively along with your desires and motivations.

Reduction Period:

If you pick out a slow approach, you can set a stop date after a reduction length. Use the time vital up to the quit date to frequently decrease the type of cigarettes you smoke each day. This technique lets in you to mentally prepare for the final prevent date.

Plan Around Stressful Periods:

Avoid choosing a quit date sooner or later of a very stressful duration, which include artwork ultimate dates or own family crises. Opt for a time at the same time as you could interest in your dedication to quitting without the added stress of outside stressors.

Consult a Healthcare Professional:

If you've got had been given health concerns or situations, are looking for for advice from a healthcare professional in advance than setting a save you date. They can provide guidance on the amazing time to cease based totally on your character health activities.

Commit to a Special Event:

Plan to take part in a very unique occasion speedy after your give up date. Knowing that you'll be attending a party, holiday, or different amusing interest can provide greater motivation to live smoke-unfastened.

Prepare and Set Goals:

Use the time fundamental up for your end date to put together mentally and set practical dreams. Establish a plan, accumulate useful useful resource, and description the benefits of quitting to preserve you focused and inspired.

Chapter 2: Building A Support System

Friends and family play a essential position in the quitting approach whilst someone is making an attempt to overcome smoking. Their resource can offer emotional encouragement, realistic assistance, and a enjoy of responsibility. Here are numerous processes in which pals and circle of relatives contribute to the success of quitting smoking:

Emotional Support:

Quitting smoking can be emotionally tough. Friends and own family can offer information, empathy, and encouragement at some point of moments of stress, frustration, or anxiety.

Accountability:

Sharing your purpose to prevent smoking with buddies and family creates a experience of obligation. Knowing that others are aware about your dedication can inspire you to stay on the proper track and face up to the urge to smoke.

Positive Reinforcement:

Friends and circle of relatives can offer effective reinforcement thru acknowledging and celebrating your achievements, no matter how small. This excellent remarks boosts self warranty and reinforces the significance of the surrender journey.

Participation in Healthy Activities:

Engaging in sports with pals and own family that don't contain smoking enables create new, smoke-unfastened routines. These sports sports can offer a distraction from cravings and promote a extra in shape lifestyle.

Communication and Understanding:

Open communication with cherished ones approximately your quitting technique lets in them to apprehend the traumatic conditions you can face. This statistics can cause a more supportive surroundings and assist keep away from capability triggers.

Offering Distractions:

Friends and circle of relatives can assist distract you all through moments of craving with the resource of venture conversations, suggesting sports activities, or sincerely being present. Distractions can redirect your cognizance away from the urge to smoke.

Participating in Quitting Programs Together:

If other circle of relatives people or buddies additionally smoke, recollect quitting together. Having a help system interior your instantaneous circle will boom the hazard of success and offers shared research.

Assistance with Stress Management:

Friends and own family can help in coping with pressure, a commonplace reason for smoking. They may additionally offer advice, lend a listening ear, or maybe participate in strain-reducing sports activities collectively.

Creating a Smoke-Free Home Environment:

If feasible, encourage those on your family to assist your efforts by means of way of retaining a smoke-free domestic. This allows dispose of triggers and reinforces the dedication to a smoke-loose way of life.

Being Non-Judgmental:

It's important for friends and family to be non-judgmental and affected man or woman. Quitting smoking is a device, and setbacks may additionally moreover arise. Having a supportive, know-how surroundings must make it simpler to navigate worrying situations.

Celebrating Milestones:

Friends and own family can actively participate in celebrating your milestones, together with the primary day with out smoking, the number one week, or the number one month. Recognition of achievements affords pleasant reinforcement.

Encouraging Professional Help:

Friends and own family can inspire looking for expert assist, which includes counseling or resource companies, and offer to accompany you to appointments or conferences.

In summary, the useful resource of friends and own family is beneficial within the quitting device. Their encouragement, information, and active involvement contribute to a incredible surroundings that complements your opportunities of correctly overcoming nicotine addiction and maintaining a smoke-free lifestyles.

Connecting with useful resource organizations and sources is a essential step in the adventure to give up smoking. These companies and assets can offer treasured statistics, encouragement, and a sense of community. Here's how you could efficaciously connect to help agencies and resources:

Online Support Communities:

Explore on line structures and boards devoted to smoking cessation. Websites, boards, and social media companies offer a area to percentage experiences, attempting to find advice, and hook up with human beings going via comparable disturbing situations.

Quitline Services:

Many nations offer quitline offerings with trained counselors who provide help over the mobile phone. These services frequently offer personalised advice, resources, and help in developing a give up plan.

National and Local Organizations:

Check with national and neighborhood health corporations for information on smoking cessation applications and assist companies. These organizations may additionally provide in-individual or digital meetings, counseling offerings, and in addition resources.

Mobile Apps:

Numerous mobile apps are designed to assist humans of their stop adventure. These apps often offer monitoring gear, motivational messages, and a community of customers sharing their evaluations. Examples consist of SmokefreeTXT and QuitGuide.

Healthcare Professionals:

Consult together with your healthcare company for steering and hints on nearby guide groups or cessation applications. They can provide custom designed recommendation, prescribe medicinal capsules if wished, and display your development.

Community Centers and Health Clinics:

Local community centers, health clinics, or hospitals may also moreover host smoking cessation applications or help businesses. Check with those centers to look inside the occasion that they provide assets or can be a part of you with relevant applications.

Employee Assistance Programs (EAP):

If applicable, inquire about smoking cessation belongings via your place of job's Employee Assistance Program. Some groups offer guide and counseling offerings to personnel searching for to cease smoking.

University Health Services:

If you're a student, college fitness offerings frequently offer assets and help for quitting smoking. They also can moreover provide counseling, institution lessons, or workshops.

Attend Workshops and Events:

Look for close by workshops or sports activities centered on smoking cessation. These gatherings can provide schooling, institution useful resource, and get proper of access to to extra sources.

Chapter 3: Creating A Quit Plan

Developing a customised method for quitting smoking is crucial for fulfillment. Every man or woman is particular, so tailoring your technique to fit your precise wishes, choices, and disturbing situations can appreciably enhance your possibilities of quitting for suitable. Here's a step-with the aid of-step guide that will help you create a custom designed quitting method:

Reflect on Your Smoking Patterns:

Identify even as, wherein, and why you smoke. Understanding your smoking conduct will help you pinpoint triggers and areas for improvement on your quitting approach.

Set a Quit Date:

Choose a significant forestall date that gives you time to put together. Consider elements like non-public milestones, strain levels, and your readiness to stop.

Create a Support System:

Share your choice to prevent with buddies, own family, and coworkers. Explain how they could assist you, and keep in mind turning into a member of a manual institution or searching out guidance from a healthcare professional.

Address Triggers:

Identify situations, emotions, or sports activities sports that reason your urge to smoke. Develop opportunity techniques for coping with those triggers, which includes taking a brief walk, training deep breathing, or conducting a present day interest.

Develop Coping Mechanisms:

Find healthy techniques to deal with strain and feelings. This can also need to include exercising, meditation, mindfulness, or speaking to a chum. Experiment with precise strategies to look what works exceptional for you.

Explore Nicotine Replacement Therapy (NRT):

Consult with a healthcare expert approximately using NRT, at the side of nicotine patches, gum, lozenges, or inhalers. NRT can assist manage withdrawal symptoms and symptoms and increase your possibilities of quitting effectively.

Create a Smoke-Free Environment:

Get rid of cigarettes, lighters, and ashtrays in your property, automobile, and place of job. Establishing a smoke-loose surroundings will reduce on the spot temptations.

Plan for Cravings:

Develop a plan for managing cravings. This could likely incorporate having wholesome snacks, carrying out physical interest, or using rest techniques. Be prepared for hard moments and recognize a manner to navigate thru them.

Reward Yourself:

Establish a gadget for profitable your self at the same time as you bought milestones on your stop adventure. Celebrate your successes with non-smoking-associated treats, in conjunction with a totally precise meal, a movie night time, or a small purchase you've been trying.

Track Your Progress:

Keep a journal or use a cellular app to track your progress. Record your triggers, successes, and any annoying conditions you encounter. Regularly reviewing your achievements can be motivating.

Stay Active:

Engage in regular physical interest. Exercise can assist manage stress, beautify mood, and distract you from cravings. Find sports you enjoy to make it a sustainable a part of your way of life.

Stay Informed:

Educate your self approximately the blessings of quitting and the risks of smoking.

Understanding the super effect on your fitness can assist your motivation.

Seek Professional Help:

If wanted, bear in mind professional useful resource, including counseling or behavioral treatment. A healthcare professional can offer custom designed techniques and address the mental additives of quitting.

Review and Adjust:

Regularly look at your technique and be open to changes. If effective strategies aren't strolling, be willing to try new strategies till you find out what works extremely good for you.

Remember, quitting smoking is a technique, and setbacks can also moreover arise. Be patient with your self and live dedicated to your motive. Adjust your method as desired, and feature amusing the progress you are making alongside the manner.

Developing Coping Mechanisms:

Deep Breathing and Relaxation Techniques:

Practice deep breathing bodily sports or revolutionary muscle relaxation to manipulate strain and anxiety, two not unusual triggers for smoking.

Physical Activity:

Engage in normal bodily interest to lessen pressure and improve temper. Exercise can be a powerful coping mechanism and a distraction from cravings.

Mindfulness and Meditation:

Learn mindfulness techniques or try meditation to live gift within the second and control cravings extra efficiently.

Healthy Snacking:

Keep healthy snacks to be had to cope with the oral fixation associated with smoking. Chew sugar-unfastened gum, snack on raw greens, or experience a bit of fruit.

Replace Habits:

Replace smoking-associated behavior with new, healthier sports. For example, take a short stroll in some unspecified time in the future of your smash in preference to smoking or find out a brand new interest to occupy some time.

Social Support:

Reach out to pals, family, or a resource agency whilst you're feeling confused or tempted to smoke. Having a useful resource tool is useful in the course of difficult moments.

Positive Affirmations:

Develop super affirmations to counter horrible thoughts and self-communicate. Remind your self of the blessings of quitting and your functionality to conquer cravings.

Create Smoke-Free Zones:

Establish smoke-free zones in your private home and automobile. This can help smash the affiliation among certain environments and smoking.

Use Nicotine Replacement Therapy (NRT):

If encouraged by the use of a healthcare expert, recollect using NRT to control cravings. NRT can provide a managed and slow cut price of nicotine intake.

Counseling or Therapy:

Consider seeking out professional counseling or remedy to deal with underlying emotional triggers and increase coping strategies tailored on your particular dreams.

Stay Hydrated:

Drink hundreds of water at some point of the day. Staying hydrated can help lessen cravings and hold you centered in your cause.

Reward Yourself:

Establish a device of rewards for staying smoke-free. Treat yourself to something a laugh even as you reach milestones in your quitting adventure.

By figuring out triggers and implementing coping mechanisms, you may navigate the annoying conditions of quitting smoking greater efficiently. Experiment with specific strategies to locate what works amazing for you, and be affected character as you increase greater wholesome conduct to update smoking.

Nicotine Replacement Therapy (NRT)

Nicotine Replacement Therapy (NRT) is a extensively used and effective technique to help people save you smoking via providing managed doses of nicotine with out the harmful chemical materials placed in tobacco smoke. Here are the numerous NRT options to be had:

Nicotine Patch:

How it in reality works: The nicotine patch is a small, adhesive patch that guarantees a non-stop, managed amount of nicotine thru the pores and pores and pores and skin into the bloodstream.

Usage: Typically worn on a clean, hairless area of the pores and pores and pores and skin, which incorporates the better arm or chest. A new patch is applied every day.

Pros: Provides a constant, regular degree of nicotine Convenient and discreet.

Nicotine Gum:

How it truly works: Nicotine gum is a chewable gum that releases nicotine on the equal time as chewed. The nicotine is absorbed through the lining of the mouth.

Usage: Chew the gum slowly after which park it some of the cheek and gum to allow nicotine absorption. Chewing releases a burst of nicotine, and the technique is repeated till the gum loses its flavor.

Pros: Allows for on-call for manage of nicotine consumption. Can be useful for coping with oral fixation.

Nicotine Lozenge:

How it virtually works: Nicotine lozenges are tough, sweet-like capsules that dissolve within the mouth, releasing nicotine.

Usage: Allow the lozenge to dissolve slowly within the mouth. It's important now not to chunk or swallow the lozenge.

Pros: Provides a discreet and transportable choice. Suitable for managing cravings discreetly.

Nicotine Nasal Spray:

How it in reality works: Nicotine nasal spray can provide a tremendous mist of nicotine into the nostrils, in which it's miles absorbed via the nasal membrane.

Usage: Administered as a nasal spray, generally in a unmarried nostril, as had to manipulate cravings.

Pros: Fast-appearing and closely mimics the quick nicotine delivery of smoking.

Nicotine Inhaler:

How it certainly works: The nicotine inhaler consists of a plastic cartridge containing nicotine. When puffed, the inhaler releases a vaporized shape of nicotine into the mouth.

Usage: Puff at the inhaler as wanted. It is used further to a cigarette.

Pros: Mimics the hand-to-mouth movement of smoking Useful for addressing behavioral elements of smoking.

Combination NRT:

How it really works: Combining one of a kind styles of NRT, together with using a patch alongside side gum or lozenges, offers a greater complete method to handling cravings.

Chapter 4: Healthy Habits

Introducing powerful manner of life adjustments is a key aspect of efficiently quitting smoking. Adopting more healthy behavior no longer exceptional permits distract from cravings but additionally contribute to everyday properly-being. Here are a few exceptional way of existence changes to endure in thoughts:

Regular Physical Exercise:

Benefits:

Improves temper and decreases pressure.

Helps manage weight gain regularly related to quitting smoking.

Distracts from cravings and gives a enjoy of achievement.

Suggestions:

Start with sports you experience, like strolling, biking, or dancing.

Aim for as a minimum one hundred and fifty mins of slight-depth exercise according to week.

Healthy Eating Habits:

Benefits:

Supports typical fitness and nicely-being.

Helps manipulate weight and prevent overeating.

Provides a exceptional awareness at some stage in moments of craving.

Suggestions:

Include masses of stop result, vegetables, entire grains, and lean proteins for your food regimen.

Stay hydrated through ingesting masses of water within the course of the day.

Mindfulness and Relaxation Techniques:

Benefits:

Reduces strain and anxiety, not unusual triggers for smoking.

Enhances self-attention and recognition on the existing 2nd.

Suggestions:

Practice mindfulness meditation or deep-respiration carrying activities.

Consider yoga or tai chi for a mixture of physical activity and mindfulness.

New Hobbies and Interests:

Benefits:

Occupies some time with exciting and high-quality sports activities.

Provides a high nice outlet for pressure and tedium.

Suggestions:

Explore new hobbies which encompass portray, gardening, cooking, or gambling a musical tool.

Join golf equipment or groups that align collectively collectively together with your pursuits.

Social Connections:

Benefits:

Provides emotional guide in some unspecified time in the future of the quitting device.

Offers a distraction from cravings via social interactions.

Suggestions:

Strengthen modern-day relationships and domesticate new ones.

Participate in social sports activities or be part of golf equipment to fulfill new human beings.

Stress Management Techniques:

Benefits:

Helps cope with strain with out resorting to smoking.

Improves cutting-edge intellectual properly-being.

Suggestions:

Practice pressure-lowering techniques in conjunction with modern-day muscle rest or guided imagery.

Consider counseling or remedy to cope with underlying stressors.

Adequate Sleep:

Benefits:

Enhances mood and cognitive feature.

Supports common health and nicely-being.

Suggestions:

Aim for 7-nine hours of fine sleep regular with night time time.

Establish a regular sleep habitual and create a comfortable sleep surroundings.

Hydration:

Benefits:

Helps manage oral cravings and keeps you hydrated.

Supports ordinary fitness and electricity.

Suggestions:

Drink water often at a few diploma inside the day.

Limit or keep away from excessive caffeine and alcohol consumption.

Education and Learning:

Benefits:

Stimulates the thoughts and fosters private growth.

Provides a incredible consciousness for highbrow power.

Suggestions:

Enroll in publications, attend workshops, or have a look at books on topics of interest.

Stay curious and open to reading new things.

Volunteering and Helping Others:

Benefits:

Creates a sense of purpose and success.

Enhances arrogance and nicely-being.

Suggestions:

Volunteer for network corporations or charitable reasons.

Offer your capabilities and time to help others in need.

Financial Planning:

Benefits:

Motivates you to keep coins formerly spent on cigarettes. -

Provides a extremely good attention on future monetary desires.

Suggestions:

Create a fee range and allocate rate range for particular goals or treats.

Consider consulting with a economic representative for customized recommendation.

Personal Development Goals:

Benefits:

Fosters a experience of personal growth and success.

Redirects strength within the course of amazing self-improvement.

Suggestions:

Set and paintings closer to private improvement desires, whether profession-related, academic, or fitness-oriented.

Celebrate achievements alongside the manner.

Remember, the key is to find sports sports and behavior that resonate with you in my opinion. Gradually incorporating these outstanding life-style changes into your each day everyday can create a fulfilling and smoke-unfastened life. It's approximately building a brand new, more wholesome manner of life that permits your well-being and allows you thrive without cigarettes.

Here are hints on vitamins, exercising, and stress control to help your popular properly-being, especially in some unspecified time in the future of the technique of quitting smoking:

Nutrition:

Hydrate Well:

Drink masses of water inside the route of the day to stay hydrated. Water allows flush out pollution and supports numerous bodily capabilities.

Eat Balanced Meals:

Include some of end result, veggies, entire grains, and lean proteins to your food. Aim for a balanced and nutritious weight loss plan.

Healthy Snacking:

Choose healthy snacks to control cravings. Options like culmination, nuts, or yogurt can be pleasant and provide essential nutrients.

Limit Caffeine and Sugar Intake:

Be aware of immoderate caffeine and sugar intake, as they could make a contribution to expanded pressure and disrupt sleep.

Consider Small, Frequent Meals:

Eating smaller, extra not unusual meals in some unspecified time in the future of the day can help stabilize blood sugar tiers and prevent overeating.

Supplement Wisely:

If wished, don't forget taking dietary supplements like vitamins and minerals to cope with any nutritional gaps. Consult with a healthcare professional for customized suggestions.

Exercise:

Start Gradually:

If you're new to exercise or haven't been lively for a while, start with low-effect sports like strolling and often boom depth.

Find Enjoyable Activities:

Choose bodily sports that you revel in to make physical hobby a sustainable a part of your routine. This may be some thing from dancing to hiking.

Mix Cardio and Strength Training:

Incorporate a aggregate of cardiovascular sports activities (e.G., on foot, on foot, cycling) and energy training to improve latest health.

Set Realistic Goals:

Set potential health dreams and tune your improvement. Celebrate small milestones to stay stimulated.

Include Flexibility Exercises:

Stretching and versatility bodily video video games, which includes yoga or Pilates, can enhance flexibility and decrease muscle anxiety.

Make It Social:

Exercise with friends or be part of company classes to make physical hobby extra a laugh and create a enjoy of community.

Prioritize Consistency:

Aim for as a minimum 100 and fifty mins of mild-intensity aerobic hobby or 75 mins of complete of lifestyles-intensity interest ordinary with week, on the facet of muscle-strengthening sports activities sports on or extra days consistent with week.

Stress Management:

Practice Deep Breathing:

Incorporate deep respiratory wearing sports to calm the worried gadget and manipulate stress. Focus on gradual, deep breaths.

Mindfulness Meditation:

Engage in mindfulness meditation to stay gift and decrease anxiety. Apps and guided commands may be beneficial for novices.

Regular Physical Activity:

Exercise is a powerful pressure reliever. Find activities you enjoy, whether or not it's strolling, on foot, swimming, or dancing.

Establish a Relaxation Routine:

Create a normal that promotes rest earlier than bedtime. This may encompass activities like studying, taking a warmth tub, or working towards rest carrying activities.

Time Management:

Prioritize obligations and set realistic desires to manage workload and avoid vain pressure. Break duties into smaller, more practicable steps.

Set Boundaries:

Learn to mention no at the same time as crucial and set up limitations to shield some time and energy.

Connect with Others:

Share your feelings with friends, circle of relatives, or a help organization. Social connections offer emotional help all through stressful instances.

Engage in Enjoyable Activities:

Make time for sports you revel in, whether or not it's a interest, spending time with loved ones, or taking element in nature. Fun and rest are essential for significant nicely-being.

Professional Support:

Consider attempting to find professional help thru counseling or remedy to observe powerful strain manipulate strategies.

Quality Sleep:

Prioritize sleep hygiene through way of growing a snug sleep environment and preserving a constant sleep schedule. Quality sleep is important for pressure manage.

Remember, those guidelines are widespread recommendations, and it's critical to tailor them for your individual alternatives and wishes. Gradually incorporating the ones practices into your every day life can contribute to higher huge fitness and help your adventure toward a smoke-unfastened lifestyle.

Chapter 5: Dealing With Cravings

Handling cravings is a crucial trouble of quitting smoking. Here are sensible strategies that will help you control and overcome cravings:

Delay and Distract:

When a yearning hits, inform yourself to count on at least 10 minutes. Use this time to interact in a distracting interest, on the facet of taking a short stroll, doing a short workout, or schooling deep breathing. Often, the yearning will skip within the course of this put off.

Deep Breathing:

Practice deep respiration carrying sports to calm your thoughts and reduce pressure. Inhale slowly through your nose, hold your breath for a few seconds, and exhale slowly thru your mouth. Repeat numerous times till you revel in greater cushty.

Positive Visualization:

Visualize a splendid picture or state of affairs that brings you pride and quietness. Close your eyes and immerse yourself on this highbrow photograph to shift your attention a long way from the craving.

Use Nicotine Replacement Therapy (NRT):

If you're using NRT, use it as directed throughout moments of excessive cravings. Nicotine opportunity can assist manipulate withdrawal symptoms and symptoms and signs and reduce the urge to smoke.

Change Your Environment:

Move to a incredible vicinity or alternate your surroundings at the same time as a yearning takes vicinity. This physical change can disrupt the association among your environment and smoking.

Oral Substitutes:

Keep oral substitutes reachable, which embody sugar-loose gum, mints, or crunchy greens. Chewing or sucking on a few element can assist satisfy the oral fixation related to smoking.

Stay Hydrated:

Drink water frequently at some point of the day. Staying hydrated can help control cravings and enhance normal well-being.

Cognitive Behavioral Techniques:

Challenge and trade terrible thoughts related to cravings. Remind your self of the motives you made a decision to end and the advantages of a smoke-loose existence.

Physical Activity:

Engage in bodily activity to distract yourself from cravings and launch endorphins, that could improve mood. A brief stroll, a hard and rapid of wearing activities, or any form of movement can be useful.

Grounding Techniques:

Use grounding strategies to deliver your self once more to the prevailing 2d. Focus at the sensations to your frame, which includes the feeling of your toes at the floor or the texture of an item to your hands.

Reach Out for Support:

Call or message a chum, member of the family, or a manual man or woman even as you're experiencing a sturdy craving. Sharing your emotions with someone supportive can offer encouragement.

Keep a Craving Journal:

Track your cravings in a magazine. Note the time, triggers, and the manner you efficiently managed the yearning. This assist you to pick out patterns and extend effective strategies.

Mindfulness Meditation:

Practice mindfulness meditation to deliver popularity on your mind and emotions with out judgment. Mindfulness can help you take a look at cravings with out giving in to them.

Positive Affirmations:

Repeat outstanding affirmations to enhance your dedication to quitting. Affirmations can assist shift your mind-set and collect self perception to your capability to face as much as cravings.

Reward Yourself:

Establish a reward tool for successfully handling cravings. Treat your self to a small reward at the same time as you triumph over a in particular tough 2nd.

Professional Support:

Consider searching out expert help through counseling or resource businesses. A counselor can offer tailor-made strategies to address cravings.

Create a Quit Kit:

Prepare a cease bundle deal with devices that convey you consolation and distraction, collectively with a stress ball, a list of motives to quit, or a favourite ebook.

Remember, cravings are quick, and with workout, the ones techniques can end up effective tools in your journey to surrender smoking. Experiment with outstanding techniques to find what works great for you, and be affected person with your self as you growth new conduct.

Mindfulness and relaxation sports can be powerful gadget to help manipulate stress, anxiety, and cravings subsequently of the approach of quitting smoking. Here are some mindfulness and rest strategies that you may contain into your every day routine:

Mindfulness Meditation:

Mindful Breathing:

Find a quiet region to sit down down with out a problem.

Focus your interest to your breath.

Inhale slowly via your nose, experience the breath getting into your lungs.

Exhale slowly through your mouth, noticing the feeling of breath leaving your frame.

Continue to interest on your breath, bringing your interest lower back if your mind starts offevolved to wander.

Body Scan Meditation:

Lie down or take a seat down down without problems.

Pay attention to every part of your body, starting out of your ft and shifting up for your head.

Notice any sensations with out judgment.

Release anxiety as you exhale.

Guided Meditation:

Listen to guided meditation intervals, which often include a narrator crucial you via relaxation physical sports activities.

Many apps and on line structures offer guided meditations for numerous skills, which encompass pressure good buy.

Relaxation Exercises:

Progressive Muscle Relaxation (PMR):

Sit or lie down in a cushty characteristic.

Tense and then progressively release every muscle group in your body, starting from your toes and operating your way up to your head.

Focus at the evaluation between anxiety and relaxation.

Visualization:

Close your eyes and consider a non violent scene, which consist of a beach, wooded area, or meadow.

Engage all of your senses within the visualization, noticing the colours, sounds, and smells.

Spend a few minutes immersed on this intellectual image.

Breath Counting:

Sit without problem together with your eyes closed.

Inhale deeply and then exhale.

Count every breath cycle, aiming to depend up to 10.

If your mind wanders, begin all another time from one.

Mindful Activities:

Eating Mindfully:

Pay near hobby to the sensory enjoy of eating.

Notice the flavors, textures, and smells of each chunk.

Chew slowly and get delight from each mouthful.

Walking Meditation:

Take a slow, aware stroll.

Pay hobby to every step, the sensation of your feet at the floor, and your breath.

Engage all of your senses in the act of strolling.

Mindful Listening:

Choose a calming piece of song or nature sounds.

Close your eyes and reputation your hobby at the sounds.

Notice each detail, from the instruments to the pauses between notes.

Quick Relaxation Techniques:

Box Breathing (4-four-4-four):

Inhale for a take into account of four.

Hold your breath for a rely of four.

Exhale for a count quantity of 4.

Pause for a count number of four.

Repeat numerous instances.

three-three-6 Breathing:

Inhale slowly for a keep in mind of 3.

Hold your breath for a remember of three.

Exhale slowly for a rely of six.

Repeat as favored.

Incorporating Mindfulness in Daily Life:

Mindful Pause:

Throughout the day, take a second to pause and convey your interest to the triumphing 2nd.

Notice your breath, the sensations for your frame, and the environment around you.

Gratitude Practice:

Take a few moments each day to reflect on belongings you're grateful for.

Write them down in a gratitude magazine.

Remember, consistency is excessive at the same time as incorporating mindfulness and rest into your normal. Experiment with special techniques and discover what resonates extraordinary with you. Regular practice can beautify your ability to stay present, manage strain, and navigate cravings more effectively.

Chapter 6: Overcoming Challenges

Quitting smoking may be a hard manner, and loads of human beings come upon various limitations alongside the way. Here are a few commonplace obstacles and techniques to address them:

Nicotine Withdrawal Symptoms:

Strategy: Nicotine alternative remedy (NRT) such as patches, gum, or lozenges can help control withdrawal symptoms and signs and symptoms. Consult with a healthcare expert to decide the most suitable desire for you.

Cravings:

Strategy: Identify triggers and increase coping techniques. Distract your self with sports sports, workout deep breathing, or chew gum at the identical time as cravings get up.

Weight Gain Concerns:

Strategy: Focus on a healthy food plan and ordinary exercising to restriction weight benefit. Keep healthy snacks on hand, and remember consulting with a nutritionist for steerage.

Social Pressure:

Strategy: Communicate with buddies and own family approximately your desire to stop. Ask for their resource and permit them to recognize how they're capable of help. Avoid situations in which you may enjoy pressured to smoke.

Emotional Triggers:

Strategy: Find possibility approaches to deal with stress, tension, or boredom. Consider sports like exercise, meditation, or carrying out pastimes to distract your self from emotional triggers.

Lack of Support:

Strategy: Join a support group, each in-character or on-line, to hook up with others who also are quitting. Share your critiques, are looking for recommendation, and provide assist to others.

Fear of Failure:

Strategy: Set realistic goals and feature an amazing time small victories. If you slip up, don't view it as a failure. Learn from the enjoy and use it as motivation to preserve your give up journey.

Routine Disruption:

Strategy: Create new sports to update smoking-associated behavior. This can help harm the affiliation among sure sports and smoking.

Negative Mood and Irritability:

Strategy: Understand that mood swings are a not unusual part of nicotine withdrawal. Practice relaxation techniques, collectively with deep respiratory or yoga, to govern stress and enhance temper.

Overconfidence:

Strategy: Recognize that quitting is an ongoing manner, and overconfidence can cause relapse. Stay vigilant, mainly in the direction of hard situations, and maintain to use the techniques which have helped you.

Boredom:

Strategy: Find new hobbies or activities to keep your self engaged. Boredom can be a purpose for smoking, so having possibility procedures to occupy it sluggish is important.

Chapter 7: Celebrating Milestones

Recognizing and worthwhile your development in quitting smoking is vital for retaining motivation and reinforcing the wonderful adjustments you're making. Here are some approaches to recognize your achievements and spotlight the blessings of a smoke-unfastened lifestyles:

Celebrate Milestones:

Set up milestones for your self, together with sooner or later, one week, one month, and so forth, and feature an super time even as you achieve them. Treat yourself to some issue particular, whether or not or not or no longer it's a fave meal, a chilled hobby, or a small praise.

Create a Reward System:

Develop a reward tool in that you allocate rewards for attaining precise goals. For example, maintain the coins you'll have spent on cigarettes and use it for something substantial, like a weekend getaway or a today's hobby.

Document Your Achievements:

Keep a mag to record your improvement. Note the effective modifications you've experienced, each bodily and emotionally. Reflecting to your achievements may be a powerful motivator.

Share Success with Others:

Share your fulfillment with buddies, family, or a guide group. Letting others understand approximately your achievements can improve yourself perception and create a nice manual tool spherical you.

Focus on Health Improvements:

Highlight the great changes for your fitness. Improved lung characteristic, better stamina, and a discounted chance of numerous ailments are massive benefits of quitting smoking. Regularly remind yourself of these fitness upgrades.

Engage in Physical Activity:

Use your advanced lung potential and power to interact in physical sports activities you enjoy. Exercise may be a wonderful manner to praise yourself even as reinforcing the incredible impact of a smoke-free manner of life on your popular nicely-being.

Treat Yourself to Self-Care:

Dedicate time to self-care sports activities that sell relaxation and nicely-being. Whether it's taking a heat bath, running closer to mindfulness, or gambling a fave hobby, prioritize sports sports that make a contribution in your intellectual and emotional health.

Educate Yourself:

Learn greater about the lengthy-time period benefits of quitting smoking. Understanding how your frame continues to heal and beautify through the years may be a effective motivator.

Save and Splurge:

Calculate the coins you've saved through the usage of not shopping for cigarettes. Consider treating your self to a few issue precise with the coins you've saved, whether or no longer or not it's a small highly-priced item or a larger purchase over the years.

Visual Reminders:

Create seen reminders of your improvement. This may be a chart tracking the instances because you surrender or a imaginative and prescient board showcasing the high fine changes you're working toward.

Connect with a Quit Buddy:

If feasible, find a cease friend or be a part of a assist group wherein you can percent and have an first-rate time milestones together. Having someone to percentage your adventure with could make the way more fun and worthwhile.

Remember that spotting progress is an ongoing method. Regularly revisit your achievements, live focused at the high excellent components of a smoke-free existence, and use those reinforcements to reinforce your willpower to quitting smoking.

Staying Quit for the Long Term

Maintaining a smoke-unfastened way of life calls for ongoing willpower and try. Here are strategies that will help you stay smoke-loose:

Build a Strong Support System:

Surround your self with supportive pals, own family, and/or a prevent-smoking assist employer. Having individuals who apprehend your adventure can provide encouragement in a few unspecified time inside the future of difficult instances.

Identify and Manage Triggers:

Recognize situations, feelings, or sports that may motive the urge to smoke. Develop possibility coping techniques to cope with those triggers, which encompass deep breathing, exercising, or undertaking a brand new interest.

Stay Active:

Regular bodily hobby can assist control pressure, beautify mood, and decrease cravings. Find sports you revel in, whether or not or now not it's strolling, taking walks, cycling, or taking aspect in a collection health beauty.

Create New Habits:

Replace smoking-related behavior with greater wholesome alternatives. For example, if you used to smoke inside the course of breaks, take a quick walk or exercise rest techniques alternatively.

Manage Stress:

Explore stress-discount techniques at the aspect of meditation, yoga, or deep breathing sports sports. Finding powerful procedures to control pressure can save you it from becoming a reason for smoking.

Rewards for Staying Smoke-Free:

Establish a reward gadget for staying smoke-loose. Treat your self to a few issue unique at unique milestones to enhance awesome behavior.

Remind Yourself of the Benefits:

Regularly replicate on the advantages of a smoke-loose life, along side advanced health, stepped forward electricity, and economic economic economic financial savings. Reminding yourself of these powerful changes could make stronger your determination.

Plan for Challenging Situations:

Anticipate conditions wherein you is probably tempted to smoke and amplify a plan to navigate them effectively. Having a method in vicinity can empower you to make extra wholesome alternatives.

Stay Informed:

Continue teaching yourself about the damaging consequences of smoking Stay knowledgeable approximately the fitness advantages you is experiencing and decorate your determination to a smoke-loose existence.

Celebrate Anniversaries:

Celebrate your smoke-loose anniversaries as a manner to recognize your accomplishments and dedication. Whether it's month-to-month or yearly, take time to famend your improvement.

Get Professional Support:

If you locate it hard to live smoke-unfastened, bear in mind searching for professional assist. Counseling, behavioral therapy, or medicinal drugs prescribed through a healthcare commercial enterprise employer can offer greater aid.

Be Patient and Persistent:

Understand that the journey to a smoke-free life is a system, and setbacks might also occur. Be affected character with your self, studies from any demanding conditions, and persist to your willpower to quit.

Engage in Activities You Enjoy:

Fill a while with sports activities you discover captivating and a laugh. This can help combat boredom and decrease the threat of turning to smoking as a manner to skip the time.

Stay Positive:

Cultivate a notable mind-set. Focus on the improvements you've made and the blessings of a smoke-loose existence in preference to dwelling on the demanding situations.

Remember, staying smoke-unfastened is a non-public adventure, and what works for one man or woman can be specific for a few different. It's crucial to find out techniques that align collectively along side your alternatives and manner of lifestyles. If you come upon difficulties, don't hesitate to are looking for for beneficial resource from healthcare professionals or smoking cessation programs.

Preventing relapse is a important detail of preserving a smoke-loose lifestyle. Here are some tips that will help you avoid returning to smoking:

Stay Connected to Support:

Maintain connections with buddies, own family, or a guide organization. Share your improvement and issues, and are seeking for support at some stage in tough instances.

Regularly Reflect on Your Reasons for Quitting:

Remind yourself of the motives why you made a decision to forestall smoking. Reflect at the fitness blessings, monetary financial financial savings, and different best modifications to your existence.

Chapter 8: Motivational Anecdotes

Here are some motivational anecdotes to encourage readers to forestall smoking:

The Clean Canvas:

Imagine your frame as a pristine canvas, and each cigarette is a stroke of darkish paint marring its splendor. Quitting smoking is like reclaiming that canvas, allowing the real shades of fitness and power to shine through. Every day without a cigarette is a brushstroke inside the direction of a greater wholesome, cleanser masterpiece.

The Phoenix's Flight:

Just because the legendary phoenix rises from its very very very own ashes, quitting smoking lets in you to emerge from the grip of cigarettes, renewed and stronger. Every day you resist the urge to smoke, you're hovering higher and reclaiming your life from the ashes of addiction.

The Butterfly's Transformation:

Like a caterpillar remodeling right right into a butterfly, quitting smoking is your metamorphosis. It might also seem tough at instances, however the forestall prevent result is a stunning, smoke-loose model of your self. Embrace the adventure of transformation, and permit your wings spread as you leave smoking in the back of.

The Symphony of Health:

Your body is like a symphony, and each organ performs a important function in growing a harmonious melody of fitness. Smoking disrupts this symphony, developing discord and disharmony. Quitting smoking permits your frame to head again to its natural us of a, where every observe contributes to the lovable composition of properly-being.

The Ocean of Well-Being:

Picture your existence as a good sized ocean of properly-being. Smoking is like throwing poisonous waste into this pristine sea, polluting it with each puff. Quitting smoking is the technique of cleansing up your ocean, restoring its purity, and allowing the waves of fitness to scrub over you.

The Garden of Life:

Consider your body as a lawn. Smoking is like weeds that choke the existence out of your beautiful vegetation. Quitting smoking is just like pulling out those weeds, permitting the vegetation of health to bloom. Nurture your lawn, and allow it flourish without the intrusion of smoking.

The Sunrise of Renewal:

Every morning with out a cigarette is a dawn of renewal. Quitting smoking is a every day possibility to start sparkling, leaving the ashes of yesterday within the again of and embracing the dawn of a extra healthy, smoke-free destiny.

The Journey Home:

Quitting smoking is like locating your way domestic after a long and arduous adventure.

With every step far from cigarettes, you're getting in the path of the warmth and luxury of a smoke-loose home. The route might be difficult, but the vacation spot is actually worth it.

Remember, each step inside the route of quitting smoking is a step in the path of a more fit, greater colorful existence. Embrace the journey, rejoice your development, and permit the anecdotes inspire you on your path to turning into smoke-loose.

Chapter 9: Understanding Smoking Addiction

Smoking addiction is a complicated interplay of physiological and behavioral elements. In this phase, we are able to delve into the complicated elements that make contributions to nicotine dependency, together with the technological information within the lower again of it, the behavioral factors that improve smoking behavior, and the significance of spotting triggers that can motive relapse.

The Science behind Nicotine Addiction

Nicotine, the primary psychoactive substance in tobacco, is a effective stimulant that acts on the mind's reward tool. When someone smokes, nicotine unexpectedly enters the bloodstream and reaches the thoughts, in which it binds to receptors, freeing neurotransmitters collectively with dopamine. Dopamine is a key participant within the thoughts's praise pathway, growing emotions of pleasure and reinforcement.

Over time, repeated exposure to nicotine leads to neuroadaptation, wherein the mind adjusts its functioning to address the presence of the drug. These version outcomes inside the improvement of tolerance, requiring human beings to smoke extra to accumulate the same fun results simultaneously, the thoughts will become extra sensitive to stress and pain inside the absence of nicotine, most important to the onset of withdrawal symptoms.

The combination of the reinforcing outcomes of nicotine and the ache of withdrawal bureaucracy a powerful cycle of dependancy Breaking this cycle involves not only addressing the bodily dependence on nicotine however additionally addressing the psychological and behavioral factors that make a contribution to the addiction.

Behavioral Aspects of Smoking

While nicotine creates a bodily dependence, the normal and ritualistic nature of smoking is in addition tremendous in keeping the addiction. Smoking frequently becomes intertwined with each day physical sports, social sports, and emotional states. Behavioral cues, which consist of the act of lighting fixtures a cigarette after a meal or at some point of a harm, come to be deeply ingrained, developing a sturdy association amongst precise conditions and the choice to smoke.

Understanding and tough those behavioral components are critical additives of a a success give up strive. Behavioral remedies, such as cognitive-behavioral remedy (CBT), interest on identifying and enhancing the mind and behaviors that make contributions to smoking. This can include growing possibility coping mechanisms for pressure, locating new workouts to update smoking triggers, and addressing the highbrow factors that perpetuate the addiction.

Recognizing Triggers

Triggers are stimuli or situations that evoke the urge to smoke, making them a massive assignment throughout the quitting method. These triggers may be various and encompass environmental cues, emotional states, social situations, or possibly specific instances of the day. Recognizing and managing triggers is essential for building resilience toward relapse.

Environmental triggers can also encompass places in which a person used to smoke or the sight of a cigarette %. Emotional triggers may be strain, tension, or possibly moments of celebration. Social triggers can also involve socializing with friends who smoke. Time-associated triggers may additionally moreover encompass the normal smoke breaks taken in the direction of particular hours.

Developing consciousness of these triggers is the first step towards powerful control. Keeping a magazine to music even as cravings occur and identifying the related triggers can provide valuable insights. Once identified, humans can work on developing strategies to navigate those triggers without resorting to smoking. This should in all likelihood contain adopting greater wholesome coping mechanisms, searching for manual from buddies and family, or distracting oneself with possibility sports activities activities.

In cease, facts smoking dependancy consists of acknowledging the complex interplay of physiological and behavioral elements. The technological know-how at the back of nicotine addiction underscores the need to address each physical dependence and intellectual factors. Behavioral factors, together with the ritualistic nature of smoking, necessitate centered interventions which include behavioral remedy alternatives. Recognizing and coping with triggers is a crucial talent for people searching to interrupt unfastened from the cycle of dependancy, enhancing the chances of a a success forestall strive.

HEALTH BENEFITS OF QUITTING SMOKING

Quitting smoking yields profound health benefits, every inside the instantaneous aftermath and over the long term. This segment explores the high brilliant changes human beings enjoy rapidly after quitting and the massive, lasting improvements that make a contribution to an trendy advanced pleasant of existence.

Immediate Changes After Quitting

The preference to give up smoking initiates a cascade of on the spot first rate adjustments inside the frame. Within only some hours, the heart charge starts offevolved offevolved to normalize, lowering the strain at the cardiovascular system. Carbon monoxide, a unstable chemical determined in cigarette smoke, decreases, allowing the blood's oxygen-carrying capability to move returned to gold favored levels.

As early as forty eight hours after quitting, the experience of taste and odor starts offevolved to get higher. Smokers often report a heightened capability to recognize flavors and smells, enhancing their popular sensory reports. Additionally, lung function starts to beautify, with improved airway dilation and decreased breathing symptoms.

In the primary few weeks, motion improves, number one to higher blood go with the float to the extremities. This is often large via warmer fingers and toes. Coughing and shortness of breath, not unusual symptoms amongst people who smoke, start to diminish because the respiration device undergoes repair.

Perhaps maximum substantially, the danger of a coronary coronary heart attack begins to mention no within simply the first 24 hours of quitting. The immediate extremely good changes underscore the body's notable resilience and potential to get higher once the damaging consequences of smoking are eliminated.

Long-Term Health Improvements

The prolonged-time period health benefits of quitting smoking expand an extended way beyond the preliminary weeks and months.

One of the most tremendous upgrades is a full-size discount in the chance of growing vital health conditions. Cardiovascular illnesses, which consist of coronary heart infection and stroke, are some of the leading reasons of lack of existence associated with smoking. By quitting, human beings drastically decrease their hazard of falling victim to those lifestyles-threatening situations.

Furthermore, the threat of developing numerous cancers, which incorporates lung, throat, and bladder most cancers, decreases over the years. The body's potential to restore broken cells and tissues improves, contributing to a decrease common most cancers risk. Respiratory health sees enduring improvements, lowering the chances of continual obstructive pulmonary illness (COPD) and different respiratory troubles.

Chapter 10: Setting Personal Goals

Setting non-public dreams is a essential step in the adventure to prevent smoking. It consists of defining precise goals and organising a realistic timeline to manual humans via the gadget. This segment delves into the importance of defining quitting goals and the practical worries concerned in setting up a timeline that aligns with non-public activities.

Defining Quitting Objectives

Defining smooth and unique quitting goals gives a roadmap for achievement. These desires characteristic benchmarks, helping people song their development and live advocated all through the quitting technique. When putting quitting goals, hold in thoughts the subsequent elements:

Cessation Method: Define the approach you can take to surrender smoking. This need to encompass cold turkey, sluggish cut price, or using smoking cessation aids together with nicotine substitute treatment or prescription medicinal pills.

Nicotine Dependence: Assess your diploma of nicotine dependence and tailor your goals because of this. Heavy those who smoke can also moreover set first-rate objectives in comparison to mild or occasional folks who smoke.

Health Milestones: Consider incorporating health-related desires into your plan. For example, you would possibly goal to reduce your coronary coronary coronary heart fee, beautify lung characteristic, or accumulate specific enhancements in not unusual properly-being.

Behavioral Changes: Recognize the behavioral elements of smoking and set desires to address them. This may additionally want to encompass identifying and changing smoking triggers, finding alternative coping mechanisms, and setting up new, extra wholesome sports.

Support Systems: If you propose to are looking for assist from pals, circle of relatives, or a assist group, encompass desires associated with constructing and utilising those resource systems.

By defining those goals, you create a personalized roadmap that aligns together along with your specific events and motivations. This clarity complements dedication and affords a tangible framework for measuring achievement.

Establishing a Realistic Timeline

Establishing a practical timeline is a essential element of purpose placing on the subject of quitting smoking. While the closing purpose is everlasting cessation, breaking down the device into potential steps may want to make the adventure more workable. Consider the following even as setting a timeline:

Short-Term Milestones: Define quick-term dreams that can be finished in the first days, weeks, and months of the quitting manner.

This might probably embody lowering the extensive sort of cigarettes smoked regular with day, abstaining for a specific duration, or efficaciously navigating tough conditions with out smoking.

Gradual Reduction vs. Cold Turkey: Decide whether or not you decide on a sluggish cut price approach or in case you are greater willing to give up cold turkey. Some people locate fulfillment in slowly reducing their cigarette consumption, at the same time as others determine on the decisiveness of quitting .

Flexibility: Be sensible approximately capability setbacks and assemble flexibility into your timeline. Quitting smoking is a journey, and surprising challenges can also arise. A bendy approach lets in for changes without feeling discouraged.

Seeking Professional Guidance: If using smoking cessation aids or searching for expert steering, encompass these into your timeline. Different strategies can also have diverse durations and require specific techniques for gradual withdrawal.

Long-Term Success: While short-time period goals are essential, furthermore set prolonged-term dreams that amplify beyond the initial weeks or months. This may contain milestones related to a 12 months of smoke-free living, achieving unique fitness upgrades, or carrying out economic economic financial savings dreams.

A properly-described timeline serves as a motivational device and lets in human beings track their development. Celebrating small victories alongside the way reinforces the commitment to the final goal of prolonged-time period smoking cessation.

In stop, placing personal desires is a foundational step in the journey to end smoking. Defining easy dreams tailored to individual activities and setting up a sensible timeline offer a hard and fast up approach that complements motivation and fulfillment. This proactive approach empowers humans to navigate the worrying conditions of quitting smoking with motive and determination.

CREATING A SUPPORT SYSTEM

Creating a sturdy assist tool is instrumental inside the way of quitting smoking. The journey to overcome nicotine addiction may be difficult, and having a community of manual enhances the possibility of fulfillment. This section explores the importance of concerning friends and circle of relatives, searching out expert manual, and becoming a member of beneficial useful resource organizations.

Involving Friends and Family

The manual of friends and family can be a powerful motivator in the quest to surrender smoking. Involving cherished ones in the technique not simplest presents emotional resource however moreover creates a community of duty. Consider the following techniques to involve friends and own family:

Open Communication: Communicate brazenly with your family about your choice to give up smoking. Share your motives for quitting, your goals, and the annoying situations you assume. This units the degree for understanding and aid.

Encouragement: Seek encouragement from buddies and family. Positive reinforcement and expressions of help can bolster your strength of will throughout difficult times. Celebrate milestones together, reinforcing the collective dedication on your success.

Identify Triggers: Work collaboratively to end up aware of capacity triggers and amplify strategies to govern them. Friends and own family can help create a smoke-unfastened surroundings and help in locating possibility sports within the course of times at the same time as cravings are probable to rise up.

Participate in Activities Together: Engage in sports that don't revolve around smoking. Shared research and new workout routines can assist smash the association among high-quality sports and smoking.

Educate Them: Help your family apprehend the challenges of nicotine dependancy. Education fosters empathy and equips them to provide greater effective resource. Share belongings or attend informational durations collectively.

Seeking Professional Support

Professional help can appreciably augment an individual's efforts to surrender smoking. Healthcare experts, collectively with clinical docs, counselors, and therapists, can provide customized steerage, evidence-based totally interventions, and scientific help. Here are key troubles while searching for professional help:

Consulting a Healthcare Professional: Schedule an appointment with a healthcare organization to speak about your choice to quit smoking. They can determine your today's health, provide custom designed advice, and prescribe medicinal pills or recommend different cessation aids if important.

Behavioral Therapy: Consider carrying out behavioral remedy with a professional counselor or therapist. Behavioral interventions, which consist of cognitive-behavioral remedy (CBT), can deal with the psychological factors of smoking and offer equipment for conduct amendment.

Pharmacological Interventions: Explore pharmacological interventions, which includes nicotine possibility treatment (NRT) or prescription medicines. These can assist control withdrawal symptoms and boom the possibilities of a fulfillment cessation.

Regular Check-Ins: Maintain everyday take a look at-ins together at the side of your healthcare business agency within the path of the quitting method. These appointments allow for ongoing assessment, modifications to the quit plan, and tracking of your normal health and development.

Joining Support Groups

Support companies provide a experience of network and shared evaluations, making them precious sources for humans on the adventure to stop smoking. Consider the following blessings of turning into a member of help organizations:

Shared Experiences: Interacting with others who're going thru similar reports fosters a revel in of camaraderie. Shared recollections, demanding situations, and successes create a supportive surroundings.

Accountability: Support corporations provide a incorporated tool of duty. Knowing that others are aware of your desires and development can function a powerful motivator to live heading within the proper direction.

Chapter 11: Identifying And Managing Cravings

Cravings are a not unusual venture within the path of the approach of quitting smoking, but powerful identification and management techniques can assist human beings navigate those moments of excessive desire for cigarettes. This section explores coping techniques for cravings, handling nicotine withdrawal signs and signs and symptoms, and incorporating healthy options to lessen cravings.

Coping Strategies for Cravings

Successfully handling cravings includes a aggregate of highbrow and behavioral strategies. By know-how triggers and adopting coping mechanisms, people can growth their resilience to cravings. Consider the following coping strategies:

Deep Breathing and Relaxation Techniques: Practice deep breathing bodily games or relaxation strategies whilst a craving movements. Focusing on your breath and calming your thoughts can help deplete the intensity of the craving.

Positive Affirmations: Use high-quality affirmations to enhance your determination to quitting. Remind yourself of the motives you selected to cease and the benefits you are already experiencing.

Distraction Techniques: Engage in activities that divert your hobby from the yearning. This should encompass going for a walk, being attentive to track, or immersing your self in a interest. The secret is to redirect your interest until the yearning subsides.

Physical Activity: Incorporate normal bodily hobby into your recurring. Exercise no longer tremendous distracts you from cravings but additionally releases endorphins, that would decorate mood and reduce strain.

Visualization: Visualize your self overcoming cravings and staying smoke-unfastened. Create highbrow photographs of a greater healthy, smoke-unfastened version of your self to enhance your willpower to the save you journey.

Delaying Gratification: When a yearning hits, decide to delaying your reaction for a hard and fast length. This do away with tactic allows time for the yearning to truely subside, empowering you to resist impulsive movements.

Mindfulness and Meditation: Practice mindfulness and meditation to domesticate reputation of the prevailing second. Mindfulness techniques let you test cravings without judgment, lowering their emotional impact.

Dealing with Nicotine Withdrawal Symptoms

Nicotine withdrawal signs and signs may be tough, however knowledge and coping with them are essential factors of the quitting gadget. Here are strategies for dealing with common withdrawal signs and symptoms:

Nicotine Replacement Therapy (NRT): Consider the use of NRT merchandise in conjunction with patches, gum, lozenges, or nasal spray. These provide a controlled dose of nicotine, helping to relieve withdrawal signs and symptoms and signs and symptoms and symptoms and symptoms whilst regularly reducing dependence.

Stay Hydrated: Drinking loads of water can help flush nicotine from your tool and alleviate a few withdrawal symptoms. It additionally facilitates with oral cravings thru offering a wholesome possibility.

Regular Meals and Snacks: Maintain a regular eating time table with balanced meals and snacks. This permits stabilize blood sugar degrees, reducing irritability and mood swings related to withdrawal.

Regular Sleep Patterns: Prioritize right sleep hygiene to cope with fatigue and irritability. Establish a steady sleep everyday, growing an environment conducive to exceptional sleep.

Physical Activity: Exercise no longer great distracts from cravings however additionally produces endorphins, that may decorate mood and alleviate withdrawal symptoms and symptoms and signs and symptoms and symptoms.

Seek Professional Support: Consult with a healthcare expert to talk approximately withdrawal signs and signs and discover pharmacological interventions if crucial. Professional steerage ensures a tailored method to dealing with character signs and symptoms.

Healthy Alternatives to Curb Cravings

Incorporating healthy alternatives can be an powerful method to lessen cravings without resorting to smoking. Consider the subsequent options:

Snacking on Healthy Foods: Keep healthful snacks on hand, which consist of culmination, vegetables, or nuts. Snacking can assist satisfy the oral fixation related to smoking.

Chew Gum or Sugar-Free Candy: Chewing gum or sucking on sugar-loose sweet offers a sensory enjoy just like smoking and may assist manage cravings.

Sip on Herbal Tea: Drinking natural tea can be a calming possibility to smoking. Choose calming kinds like chamomile or peppermint to assist ease pressure and cravings.

Stay Active: Engage in bodily sports activities activities that keep your hands and mind occupied. This want to consist of gardening, knitting, or each different interest that calls for guide dexterity.

Use Nicotine-Free Products: Consider using nicotine-loose options like natural cigarettes or electronic cigarettes without nicotine. These mimic the behavioral factor of smoking without the addictive substance.

Practice Aromatherapy: Use scents like essential oils or natural incense to create a pleasant environment. Certain scents, which includes lavender or citrus, can help reduce stress and cravings.

In quit, identifying and dealing with cravings is a critical element of the quitting technique. By the use of coping techniques, addressing withdrawal signs and symptoms, and incorporating wholesome alternatives, human beings can beautify their ability to triumph over cravings and navigate the demanding conditions of quitting smoking efficiently.

ADOPTING A HEALTHY LIFESTYLE

Embracing a wholesome lifestyle is crucial to the success of smoking cessation. Beyond quitting smoking, adopting terrific behavior contributes to everyday nicely-being and resilience in competition to relapse. In this section, we're able to find out the significance of incorporating exercise into your habitual, balancing nutrients for smoking cessation, and information the placement of sleep in the quitting way.

Incorporating Exercise into Your Routine

Regular exercise performs a pivotal role in smoking cessation by using way of the usage of offering bodily, highbrow, and emotional advantages. Here's why incorporating workout into your regular is critical:

Stress Reduction: Exercise is a effective strain reliever. It lets in regulate stress hormones, together with cortisol, and stimulates the manufacturing of endorphins, that are natural mood enhancers. As strain is a common cause for smoking, managing stress through exercise may be a key technique.

Craving Reduction: Physical interest has been showed to reduce cravings for cigarettes. Engaging in slight-depth sports like brisk walking, strolling, or biking can distract from cravings and reduce their intensity.

Weight Management: Some human beings can also moreover revel in weight benefit after quitting smoking. Regular exercise can beneficial resource in weight management via the usage of burning power and supporting a healthy metabolism.

Improved Lung Function: As lung characteristic improves in the path of smoking cessation, incorporating cardio sports can similarly enhance breathing capability and ordinary lung fitness.

Positive Routine Replacement: Establishing a contemporary ordinary centered spherical exercise can update the vintage smoking-associated sporting events. This exceptional substitution reinforces the dedication to a greater healthful way of life.

Social Engagement: Participating in employer physical sports or sports fosters social engagement, offering a supportive network that can inspire and encourage individuals on their cease adventure.

Whether it's far cardio physical video games, power training, or sports activities activities like yoga, finding an exercising habitual that aligns with private alternatives enhances the danger of lengthy-time period success in smoking cessation.

Balancing Nutrition for Smoking Cessation

Nutrition performs a essential role in assisting the frame's restoration method in a few unspecified time within the future of smoking cessation. Adopting a nicely-balanced and nutritious weight loss program gives severa advantages:

Support for Detoxification: Certain elements useful useful resource within the cleansing machine through promoting the elimination of pollutants associated with smoking. These encompass fruits, greens, and substances rich in antioxidants.

Stress Management: Nutrient-dense factors, along with whole grains, surrender quit result, and veggies, make a contribution to traditional nicely-being and can assist control pressure – a not unusual trigger for smoking.

Hydration: Staying successfully hydrated is vital in a few unspecified time inside the future of smoking cessation. Water enables flush pollution from the body and might assist in coping with oral cravings with the beneficial aid of providing a healthful opportunity to smoking.

Snacking Strategies: Choose wholesome snacks to manipulate oral cravings. Options like carrot sticks, nuts, or glowing fruit offer a fulfilling crunch and assist fight the hand-to-mouth addiction associated with smoking.

Balanced Meals: Ensure that food are properly-balanced, incorporating an entire lot of food companies. Balanced meals contribute to stable blood sugar stages, decreasing irritability and mood swings related to nicotine withdrawal.

Vitamin and Mineral Intake: Smoking can expend certain vitamins and minerals within the frame. A diet regime wealthy in end result, vegetables, and whole grains can help top off the ones essential nutrients. Working with a nutritionist or healthcare professional can offer personalised guidance on nutritional selections tailored to man or woman wishes and desires within the path of smoking cessation.

The Role of Sleep in Quitting

Quality sleep is a foundational detail of ordinary fitness and well-being, and it performs a outstanding feature inside the quitting way. Consider the subsequent reasons why prioritizing sleep is crucial for a hit smoking cessation:

Stress Reduction: Quality sleep is crucial for pressure reduction. Adequate rest promotes emotional resilience and permits manage strain tiers, lowering the threat of turning to cigarettes as a coping mechanism.

Improved Mood and Mental Clarity: Lack of sleep can contribute to mood swings, irritability, and trouble concentrating – common demanding situations in the route of smoking cessation. Prioritizing sleep enhances mood and cognitive function.

Chapter 12: Behavioral Changes For Smoking Cessation

Behavioral modifications are at the middle of a achievement smoking cessation. Breaking smoking conduct, adopting strain control strategies, and incorporating mindfulness and meditation into each day existence are essential additives of this transformative journey. In this section, we'll discover the importance of these behavioral adjustments and the way they make contributions to a smoke-unfastened manner of lifestyles.

Breaking Smoking Habits

Breaking the cycle of smoking conduct is a critical element of behavioral trade ultimately of the quitting device. Smoking is often intertwined with numerous sports activities sports, environments, and feelings, growing a complicated net of triggers. Consider the following strategies for breaking smoking conduct:

Identifying Triggers: Recognize situations, emotions, or sports that reason the preference to smoke This popularity is the first step in breaking the affiliation among the ones triggers and smoking.

Creating New Routines: Replace smoking-related exercises with new, extra healthful conduct For example, if you used to smoke all through breaks, recollect taking a brisk stroll or running closer to deep respiratory sports activities as an possibility.

Changing Environments: Modify environments associated with smoking. This might likely contain rearranging furnishings, repurposing smoking areas, or preserving off locations wherein smoking is permitted.

Behavioral Therapy: Engage in behavioral therapy, which include cognitive-behavioral therapy (CBT), to cope with the underlying thoughts and behaviors related to smoking. Therapeutic interventions can provide device for converting behavior and growing coping mechanisms.

Rewarding Positive Behavior: Implement a reward device for reaching milestones in your smoke-unfastened journey. Celebrate successes, whether or now not big or small, to decorate remarkable behavioral modifications.

Breaking smoking conduct is an ongoing technique that calls for staying power, willpower, and a proactive technique to reshaping one's every day exercises and behaviors.

Stress Management Techniques

Stress is a common cause for smoking, and developing effective strain manage strategies is crucial for maintaining a smoke-unfastened way of life. Consider the following pressure control techniques:

Deep Breathing Exercises: Practice deep breathing carrying activities to promote rest and reduce strain. Deep, sluggish breaths can spark off the frame's rest reaction, counteracting the physiological consequences of stress.

Physical Activity: Regular physical hobby is a effective pressure reducer. Engage in sports you enjoy, whether or not it's far taking walks, running, yoga, or dancing. Exercise releases endorphins, which decorate mood and reduce pressure.

Time Management: Efficiently manage it gradual to reduce feelings of overwhelm. Prioritize duties, set practical dreams, and smash massive obligations into smaller, potential steps.

Mindfulness Techniques: Incorporate mindfulness techniques, which incorporates mindful breathing or body scanning, into your each day recurring. Mindfulness lets in you live gift, decreasing anxiety approximately the destiny and stress approximately the past.

Relaxation Techniques: Explore rest strategies like progressive muscle relaxation or guided imagery. These strategies can activate a country of rest, assuaging pressure and tension.

Social Support: Seek assist from buddies, family, or manual organizations sooner or later of traumatic instances. Talking to others approximately your feelings can offer emotional comfort and a clean mindset on demanding situations.

Effectively managing pressure entails a aggregate of self-attention, proactive coping techniques, and a willingness to conform to lifestyles's annoying conditions with out turning to smoking as a coping mechanism.

Mindfulness and Meditation

Mindfulness and meditation are effective equipment for cultivating recognition, lowering strain, and fostering a balanced mind-set. Incorporating those practices into each day lifestyles can drastically make a contribution to smoking cessation. Consider the following approaches mindfulness and meditation can assist your journey:

Mindful Smoking: If you pick out to smoke, exercise aware smoking. Be sincerely present inside the path of the act, listening to the taste, perfume, and sensations. This aware method can create consciousness throughout the dependancy and its effect.

Guided Meditation: Utilize guided meditation training targeted on smoking cessation Many sources offer unique guided meditations designed to help humans of their adventure to prevent smoking.

Body Scan Meditation: Practice body test meditations to domesticate recognition of physical sensations. This can assist people grow to be more attuned to their our our bodies, making it less complex to emerge as aware about and deal with cravings.

Staying Present: Mindfulness encourages staying present within the 2d, reducing tension approximately the destiny or regret approximately the beyond. This may be specially beneficial at some degree in the hard moments of quitting.

Incorporating mindfulness and meditation into your regular requires consistency and a willingness to discover terrific practices. These techniques offer treasured device for dealing with cravings, growing self-recognition, and growing a extra healthy mind-set in the context of smoking cessation.

In give up, behavioral changes are pivotal in the journey to end smoking. Breaking smoking behavior, adopting strain manipulate strategies, and incorporating mindfulness and meditation contribute to a holistic approach to behavioral transformation. These modifications no longer pleasant assist smoking cessation but additionally sell substantial properly-being, resilience, and personal growth.

UTILIZING NICOTINE REPLACEMENT THERAPIES

Nicotine alternative remedy alternatives (NRTs) are precious gear in the adventure to quit smoking via supplying controlled doses of nicotine without the dangerous substances located in tobacco smoke. This phase explores the numerous NRT alternatives available, publications on deciding on the proper approach, and considerations for combining treatments for more potent effectiveness.

Overview of Nicotine Replacement Options

Nicotine replacement recovery strategies are to be had in severa forms, each designed to cope with awesome elements of nicotine dependence. Here is an define of common NRT options:

Nicotine Patch: The patch is a transdermal gadget that offers a everyday, controlled dose of nicotine thru the skin. It is normally worn at the top frame and provides a continuous release of nicotine within the path of the day.

Nicotine Gum: Nicotine gum is a chewable form of NRT that permits for on-name for nicotine intake. It is to be had in diverse strengths, and customers chew the gum to launch nicotine, this is then absorbed thru the lining of the mouth.

Nicotine Lozenge: Similar to the gum, the lozenge is a discreet and portable NRT preference. Users let the lozenge dissolve inside the mouth, freeing a controlled quantity of nicotine.

Nicotine Nasal Spray: The nasal spray affords a fast dose of nicotine thru the nasal mucosa. It offers a quicker onset of consolation in comparison to top notch NRT strategies.

Nicotine Inhaler: The inhaler is a tool that lets in customers to inhale vaporized nicotine. It mimics the hand-to-mouth motion of smoking and gives a controlled dose of nicotine.

Nicotine Sublingual Tablet: Placed underneath the tongue, the sublingual tablet dissolves to release nicotine immediately into the bloodstream thru the mucous membranes.

Choosing the proper NRT depends on character opportunities, manner of lifestyles, and the quantity of nicotine dependence. Consulting with a healthcare expert can assist determine the most suitable choice.

Choosing the Right Method for You

Selecting the right NRT approach consists of thinking about personal opportunities, way of existence elements, and the extent of nicotine dependence. Here are key issues for selecting the proper NRT method:

Daily Routine: Consider how well a selected NRT approach aligns along side your each day habitual. For folks that pick a fixed-it-and-neglect about-it approach, the patch may be appropriate. On the possibility hand, those who desire on-call for treatment may additionally moreover pick out gum, lozenges, or inhalers.

Degree of Nicotine Dependence: The degree of nicotine dependence will have an effect on the choice of NRT strength. Heavy people who smoke may additionally furthermore choose higher-dose patches or gum, on the same time as lighter individuals who smoke may also pick out decrease-dose alternatives.

Oral Fixation: Individuals who pass over the hand-to-mouth motion of smoking can also moreover find out gum, lozenges, or inhalers useful, as they mimic this element of the smoking addiction.

Convenience and Discreetness: Consider the benefit and discreetness of the selected NRT. Patches, for instance, are discreet and require minimal hobby for the duration of the day, whilst gum and lozenges provide portability.

Potential Side Effects: Be privy to capacity facet effects associated with every NRT choice. For instance, a few humans can also additionally moreover experience infection with the nasal spray, whilst others may also additionally furthermore find out consolation without terrible outcomes.

Health Considerations: Individuals with superb health situations must communicate with a healthcare professional earlier than deciding on an NRT technique. Pregnant women and people with cardiovascular issues, as an example, can also require specialised steerage.

It's critical to word that the effectiveness of NRTs is frequently maximized whilst used as part of a whole smoking cessation plan that consists of behavioral strategies and manual.

Combining Therapies for Enhanced Effectiveness

Combining unique NRT techniques can decorate effectiveness via addressing multiple elements of nicotine dependence. This method, called combination treatment, might also moreover involve using an extended-acting NRT, together with a patch, to offer a steady baseline of nicotine and a quick-performing NRT, on the side of gum or lozenges, to cope with leap forward cravings.

Consider the following advantages of aggregate remedy:

Flexible Relief: Combination remedy lets in for bendy and on-call for treatment by way of way of the use of the usage of brief-appearing

NRTs throughout moments of heightened cravings whilst maintaining a non-forestall baseline with lengthy-appearing NRTs.

Increased Quit Rates: Studies have verified that mixture treatment is regularly more effective than the usage of a unmarried NRT technique on my own. It addresses each the persistent detail of nicotine dependence and the extreme cravings that would upward thrust up.

Tailored Approach: Combination remedy allows people to tailor their technique to quitting primarily based on their precise goals and picks.

Reduced Side Effects Using decrease doses of multiple NRTs can also reduce the risk of component outcomes associated with higher doses of a single NRT.

It's essential to visit a healthcare expert earlier than embarking on aggregate treatment to make certain that the chosen techniques are well matched and safe for character fitness situations.

In conclusion, the usage of nicotine replacement treatment plans cans extensively useful resource within the tool of quitting smoking. Understanding the available options, deciding on the proper approach based totally on non-public alternatives, and thinking about combination remedy can enhance the effectiveness of NRTs as part of a complete smoking cessation plan.

Chapter 13: Dealing With Relapses

Experiencing a relapse in smoking cessation can be disheartening, but it's far critical to view it as a analyzing opportunity and an possibility to refine your technique. This segment explores know-how relapse triggers, developing a relapse prevention plan, and getting lower again on route after a relapse.

Understanding Relapse Triggers

Understanding the triggers that make contributions to relapse is essential for developing effective prevention techniques. Relapse triggers can be severa and can encompass:

Stress: High stages of stress may be a large cause for relapse. It's important to expand opportunity pressure manipulate strategies to cope with tough situations.

Social Situations: Being in conditions in which others are smoking or feeling social pressure to smoke can reason relapse. Creating a smoke-free social network and having a plan for such conditions is critical.

Emotional States: Certain emotional states, including unhappiness, anger, or boredom, can motive the desire to smoke. Developing coping mechanisms to deal with those emotions with out resorting to smoking is essential.

Habitual Triggers: Certain sports or exercises associated with smoking, which includes having a cup of espresso or taking a ruin, can motive cravings. Identifying and breaking these institutions is vital for a success cessation.

Overconfidence: Feeling overly confident approximately one's ability to stay smoke-unfastened can also purpose complacency. It's essential to stay vigilant and constantly beautify great behaviors.

Developing a Relapse Prevention Plan

Creating a relapse prevention plan is a proactive method to anticipate and address capacity disturbing situations. Here are key additives of a relapse prevention plan:

Identify Triggers: Reflect on your preceding smoking styles and pick out the triggers that brought approximately relapse. Awareness of those triggers is the first step in prevention.

Alternative Coping Strategies: Develop opportunity coping techniques for managing stress, coping with feelings, and dealing with everyday triggers. This should consist of deep respiration wearing activities, project physical interest, or searching out social useful resource.

Build a Support System: Strengthen your manual tool through concerning pals, own family, or aid businesses. Communicate your dreams and enlist their assist in instances of difficulty.

Regular Check-Ins: Schedule regular take a look at-ins with a healthcare professional or a smoking cessation counselor. These take a look at-ins offer an opportunity to talk approximately challenges, adjust your plan, and collect steering.

Set Realistic Goals: Establish practical and manageable dreams. Break down the quitting technique into ability steps, celebrating small victories alongside the way.

Learn from Previous Attempts: Reflect on beyond attempts to give up smoking. Identify what labored properly and what's going to be stepped forward. Use this understanding to refine your cutting-edge method.

Adapt to Challenges: Life is dynamic, and demanding situations are inevitable. Be prepared to comply your plan as desired. Flexibility is a key element of a fulfillment relapse prevention.

Getting Back on Track After a Relapse

Experiencing a relapse would no longer symbolize failure however rather an opportunity to expect once more and readjust your technique. Here's a manner to get once more at the proper track after a relapse:

Self-Reflection: Reflect at the times that brought about the relapse. Understanding the triggers and activities can help you develop more effective techniques moving ahead.

Avoid Self-Blame: Be compassionate with your self and keep away from self-blame. Quitting smoking is a tough method, and setbacks are a commonplace a part of the journey.

Recommit to Quitting: Reaffirm your dedication to quitting smoking. Remind your self of the reasons you decided to stop and the advantages you aspire to accumulate.

Seek Support: Reach out to your useful aid device, whether or no longer or no longer it is friends, circle of relatives, or a assist institution. Share your enjoy, and are searching for encouragement and steering.

Adjust Your Plan: Evaluate your initial end plan and make essential changes. Consider incorporating new coping strategies, addressing more triggers, or enhancing your goals.

Learn from the Experience: Use the relapse as a gaining knowledge of experience. Understand the factors that contributed to it and use this recognize-a way to beautify your relapse prevention plan.

Celebrate Progress: Acknowledge any improvement you made within the direction of your smoke-unfastened length. Celebrate the exquisite adjustments you professional and use them as motivation for the destiny. Returning to a smoke-free lifestyle after a relapse requires resilience, self-pondered photograph, and a dedication to analyzing from the enjoy. By enforcing a well-considered relapse prevention plan and seeking ongoing guide, people can navigate the disturbing situations of smoking cessation greater successfully.

CELEBRATING MILESTONES AND SUCCESSES

Recognizing and celebrating milestones and successes is a important element of the adventure to prevent smoking. It no longer exceptional offers fantastic reinforcement however also boosts motivation and reinforces the strength of will to a smoke-free life. This phase explores the importance of spotting achievements and indicates rewards for engaging in milestones.

Recognizing Achievements

Celebrating achievements, no matter how small, is important for keeping motivation and a effective attitude within the path of the smoking cessation journey. Here are strategies to understand and have an amazing time achievements:

Set Clear Milestones: Establish clear, achievable milestones alongside the manner. Whether it's far a day, each week, a month, or a specific behavioral purpose, having defined milestones lets in for normal celebrations.

Reflect on Progress: Take time to mirror at the development made because of the truth quitting smoking. Consider improvements in health, adjustments in conduct, and the overall brilliant effect on well-being.

Share Successes with Others: Share your successes with friends, own family, or a assist organisation. Celebrating with others creates a experience of network and reinforces the awesome factors of the quitting tool.

Keep a Journal: Maintain a journal to file your achievements and reflections. Documenting your adventure permits you to look returned and notice how a long way you've come, serving as a supply of motivation.

Reward Yourself: Treat your self to rewards even as carrying out specific milestones. This can be a effective motivator and reinforces the wonderful behavior of staying smoke-unfastened.

Express Gratitude: Take a 2nd to express gratitude for the aid acquired from pals, circle of relatives, or experts. Acknowledging the location of others on your fulfillment fosters a experience of connection and gratitude.

Visual Reminders: Create seen reminders of your achievements. This may be a calendar in that you mark each smoke-unfastened day or a visible instance of your development.

Rewards for Milestones

Rewarding your self for accomplishing milestones adds a high quality and exciting element to the quitting approach. Consider the subsequent thoughts for rewards at one among a type degrees of your smoke-loose adventure:

Small Daily Rewards: For each smoke-loose day, deal with your self to a small reward, which incorporates a favourite snack, a relaxing interest, or a short harm.

Weekly Treats: Set weekly dreams and praise yourself at the surrender of every successful week. This need to encompass going to a film, enjoying a completely unique meal, or indulging in a interest you like.

Monthly Celebrations: Celebrate month-to-month milestones with extra large rewards. Consider a day revel in, a spa day, or shopping for a few component you've got got been searching.

Health and Wellness Rewards: Allocate rewards that contribute on your mounted health and properly-being. This ought to include making an funding in a health tracker, joining a gymnasium or fitness elegance, or treating yourself to a health retreat.

Financial Savings: Use the cash stored from now not attempting to find cigarettes as a foundation for economic rewards. Treat your self to a few factor you've got been saving for or make contributions to a completely unique fund for a larger praise down the street.

Experience-Based Rewards: Consider experience-based totally completely rewards, along with a weekend getaway, attending a live overall performance or occasion, or collaborating in an interest you have got continually desired to strive.

Social Rewards: Share your achievements with buddies and family and plan social rewards. This might also moreover want to encompass a celebratory dinner with cherished ones or web website hosting a smoke-loose accumulating.

Educational Rewards: Invest for your personal or expert improvement as praise This need to involve enrolling in a course, attending a workshop, or exploring a trendy location of hobby.

Customize your rewards primarily based to your alternatives and hobbies, ensuring that they align on the facet of your trendy goals and make a contribution to the immoderate quality momentum of your smoking cessation journey.

In give up, celebrating milestones and successes is a essential element of the smoking cessation method. Recognizing achievements, sharing successes, and profitable oneself contribute to a effective mind-set, extended motivation, and a sustained determination to a smoke-free lifestyle.

Chapter 14: The Disconcerting Beginning

Well, right here we are. Have you observed how some choices, irrespective of how small they'll appear, may be the prelude to something big in our lives? Think approximately this: how usually have you ever attempted to surrender smoking? No, seriously, pause and think about it. Now, how pretty a few the ones times have you ever been knowledgeable that all you want is electricity of will? Or perhaps which you ought to use nicotine patch, or possibly gum, or worse, a few different shape of alternative for the act of smoking?

Now, if those strategies had been as effective as advertised, why are we right here? Why is smoking although a international epidemic, costing plenty and hundreds of lives and billions of dollars every 365 days? Have you ever wondered if possibly, certainly possibly, the set up technique for quitting smoking is incomplete, or worse, incorrect?

Let's dive into why conventional techniques of smoking cessation have failed almost across the board. Be warned: this isn't a leisurely walk thru the nicely-trodden paths of anti-smoking techniques. We are proper here to discover, question, and positive, mission the reputation quo. We're here to dig into why the well-known techniques you have got got been advised you want to have a look at religiously might not, in truth, be the Holy Grail you have were given been looking for. Dare to question, because of the fact that interest is precisely the engine on the way to pressure this transformative journey.

The truth is that conventional smoking cessation strategies are too one-dimensional. They recognition, almost exclusively, at the bodily act of smoking: take the cigarette from your hand and, voila, hassle solved! But, as you nicely realise, tobacco addiction is lots more complex. It's a tangled web that reaches into the interstices of your thoughts, your emotions, or maybe your identification. Can a nicotine patch untangle that tangled net?

Don't get us incorrect, we are not actually discrediting conventional strategies In fact, for some people, they art work. But here's the crux of the problem: what works for one doesn't constantly artwork for all and sundry. Oh, and by way of the way, have you ever ever ever tried to stop smoking handiest to discover yourself desperate for each one in all a kind shape of release, like overeating or maybe biting your nails to the fast? You're no longer the handiest one. This phenomenon is what Allen Carr dubbed as "The Great Tobacco Delusion" in his e book posted in 1985. Carr argues that dependancy is going beyond tobacco itself; it's miles a mental and emotional warfare. And you can't win a war on a couple of fronts with actually one kind of ammunition, are you capable of?

So, in case you've ever felt like a hamster on a wheel, on foot around getting nowhere on your attempts to cease smoking, you are not on my own. And most significantly, it is now not your fault.

So, pricey reader, take a deep breath (fast it's going to probable be an entire lot cleaner air, I promise) and get prepared for a whole new approach. In the chapters that look at, we're going to shake the tree of tobacco dependancy data and notice what end result fall. Some could be candy, a few bitter, however all is probably essential in your transformation.

I invite you to permit bypass of your preconceptions and open your mind. What follows will not simplest loose you from smoking, however may additionally even take you on a adventure of self-expertise and personal boom. Are you ready for this transcendental adventure? Ready to rediscover who you are with out that cloud of smoke clouding your vision and your life? Read on, because what follows is a adventure like no different. And I promise you, with the resource of the surrender of this journey, you may no longer high-quality prevent smoking, however you becomes a whole new edition of yourself.

Shall we begin?

If you're here, it's miles because of the fact you've got observed out that tobacco dependancy is not quite an lousy lot chemical compounds, nicotine, or certainly averting lighting up. As Judith Wrubel talked about in her ebook "The Dynamics of Behavior Development" (1979), addiction is a complex interplay maximum of the individual and his or her surroundings. It is some factor that is deeply rooted in our psyche, our belief system and our feelings.

One issue that many conventional techniques do not cope with is the complex interaction amongst our mind and frame in addiction. As Gabor Maté defined in "In the Realm of Hungry Ghosts: Close Encounters with Addiction" (2008), addiction is more than a rely number form of neurochemistry; it is also a rely of emotional ache, trauma, and interpersonal relationships. You can't really tear off the top leaf of this multilayered onion and anticipate all the scent to move away.

You must peel away layer after layer, dealing with every one especially and strategically.

So positive, traditional strategies can be one piece of the puzzle, however they're honestly no longer the complete photo. This turns into particularly applicable on the identical time as we're faced with the unfastened fall that follows most prevent attempts. You've been there, right? At first, everything is new and thrilling. You enjoy powerful, charged with purpose. But then, after a while, you start to be aware that a few component is lacking. Maybe it's far a feel of emptiness, possibly an unexplained urgency. It's as despite the fact that a bit of the puzzle is missing. And what are we able to do while we can't discover that missing piece? Exactly, we cross lower lower back to antique conduct, because of the reality at the least they may be acquainted.

It's thrilling how Malcolm Gladwell, in "The Tipping Point: How Small Changes Can Make Big Effects" (2000), factors out that every so often, inside the unfold of traits, behaviors or mind, we advantage what he calls "The Tipping Point" - that magic 2nd whilst an concept, fashion or conduct crosses a threshold and starts offevolved offevolved to spread like wildfire. What if we may also need to find that tipping element in our efforts to cease smoking - that thing in which it all makes experience, in which the portions of the puzzle in the end healthy together?

To find out that tipping point, you should be inclined to check the middle ideals that gasoline your addiction The strength of beliefs in conduct modification is a few aspect Tony Robbins has noted appreciably in his seminars and in his ebook "Power Without Limits" (1986). He argues that our ideals have the functionality to make or smash, and at the identical time as you may alternate one center notion, you could exchange an entire lifestyles trajectory.

So, it's time to ask you some difficult questions. What underlying ideals are using your dependency? Are they in truth yours, or are they the voices of society, pals, or perhaps the tobacco agency talking through you? As you start to remedy these questions, you prepare for the subsequent financial ruin of this journey, wherein we can delve into how tobacco takes over your mind on a neurochemical degree.

In the stop, what we're doing right right here is greater than quitting smoking; we're project an in depth restructuring of your psyche and your life. If you have got made it this a protracted way, I congratulate you. You are showing a stage of self-discipline and self-meditated picture that maximum people by no means gain. And that, my high priced reader, isn't always any small thing.

I encourage you to maintain going, because of the truth what follows is each eye-starting and releasing. Are you prepared to preserve to get to the lowest of the mysteries of your dependancy and, within the technique, discover components of yourself that you did not even understand existed? Because I promise you, whilst you reach the give up of this adventure, the individual that will emerge can be a person stronger, wiser and, truely, unfastened.

So proper right here we are, on this fascinating adventure, exploring the depths of our psyche and unraveling the strings which have positive our will to tobacco But what if I knowledgeable you that there are humans who have prevent smoking without resorting to patches, lozenges or nicotine opportunity treatment? What if I informed you that they did it virtually with the useful resource of changing their mind-set?

Here is a concrete example that can vividly illustrate this factor: Imagine you are a sailor and also you find out your self on a deliver stuck in a fierce hurricane. The winds are roaring, the waves are crashing, and the deliver's hull is creaking menacingly. In this situation, your cigarette is like an anchor which you assume is keeping you constant. But what you do not see is that the anchor has grow to be entangled in a web of debris underwater, endangering the complete deliver. In an act of bravery or possibly desperation, you decide to reduce the anchor rope. The deliver, now freed, can sail more with out trouble thru the stormy waters to calm. This easy however massive act of slicing the rope changes your destiny.

This is an example of what Charles Duhigg explores in his e-book "The Power of Habit: Why We Do What We Do in Life and Business" (2012). According to Duhigg, conduct art work in a 3-element circuit: the signal, the normal and the praise. Changing a addiction involves identifying the sign and the praise after which substituting a new habitual. Sounds easy, proper? But, right here comes the name of the game factor: notion. Without a actual perception within the possibility of change, you could relapse. So the question now is, do you be given as actual with you can exchange?

The success reminiscences of those who have efficaciously surrender smoking often revolve spherical this shift in mindset, this spark of belief. Take Sarah, a girl who had smoked for additonal than 20 years. Her recreation changer got here now not with a modern shape of nicotine patch, but at the equal time as her 5-3 hundred and sixty 5 days-vintage son handed her a drawing of the circle of relatives that showed everybody smiling, except for her, who have emerge as drawn with a cigarette and a unhappy face. This modified into a 2nd of revelation for Sarah. What type of instance modified into she putting for her son? What form of legacy did she want to go away? It modified into at that 2nd that the notion that she ought to and need to alternate lit up like a beacon in her mind. From that day on, each time she felt the urge to smoke, she might have a have a look at that drawing. She remembered her "why," and it gave her the power to face as much as.

Another author who talks about the power of attitude exchange is Viktor Frankl in his e-book "Man's Search for Meaning" (1946). Frankl, a psychiatrist and Holocaust survivor, argues that at the equal time as we cannot manipulate all the sports round us, we continuously have the energy to pick our reaction to them. In the context of quitting smoking, because of this that you constantly have the selection of the way to react on the identical time as confronted with a smoking cue.

If you've got made it this some distance, you are preparing yourself to method this adventure from a strong and properly-knowledgeable basis, armed now not handiest with tool but moreover with the proper motivation and mind-set. I congratulate you on having come this a protracted way, and I guarantee you that the journey turns into even greater captivating and enlightening from proper right right here. A deep abyss of discovery awaits us inside the next financial catastrophe, in which we're capable of explore how the mind turns into the unwitting accomplice in our dependancy to tobacco. Are you prepared to hold? Because, keep in mind me, you could no longer need to overlook what comes next.

But there you've got were given the crucial component: a changed mind-set, a modern-day thoughts-set, may need to make the act of quitting smoking a journey of self-discovery, in location of an ordeal complete of struggling.

Now, allow's be sincere: change isn't always easy. As Albert Einstein as soon as said, "We cannot resolve our issues with the equal thinking that created them." If you're seeking out a miracle, be warned, quitting smoking isn't a feat you can accomplish with the magic wand. But you could do it with the "electricity of conscious goal," as Wayne Dyer calls it in his ebook "The Power of Intention" (2004). This power is not an external pressure, but an internal pressure inside you that you may mobilize to create actual change on your existence.

It's time to alternate the narrative. You are not a prisoner of your behavior; you're the architect of your future. Can you sense how this mindset alters your mind chemistry? Can you enjoy the opportunities enlarge earlier than you?

Let me percentage a hint delusion that possibly illustrates this in a extra playful manner. Imagine you are a fish swimming in the ocean, and you have had been given commonly had a stone tied to your fin. This stone is your cigarette. Now, what ought to display up if you have been to put off that stone? At first, you may enjoy some resistance, even emptiness. But then, , you apprehend that you may swim quicker, farther, with less try. The ocean now will become a vicinity of freedom and exploration, in region of limitations. That's lifestyles without cigarettes: an ocean of possibilities.

We've covered numerous floor, no question approximately it. From statistics why conventional smoking cessation techniques won't be effective to exploring how mind-set and mindset can be our top notch allies in this journey. The horizon is plain and navigation seems less arduous while one is armed with the proper form of statistics and thoughts-set.

If you have made it this a ways, congratulations You have already taken the most essential first step: you have got were given began to expect seriously and deeply about your dating with tobacco and are prepared to take manage. Don't forget about that you aren't on my own on this journey; we are right here to sail those seas together.

In the following bankruptcy, get your neurons organized for a intellectual gymnastics session, as we are going to input the charming neural highways of your thoughts. We'll cope with how tobacco without a doubt "hijacks" your mind, and no, it genuinely is no longer a euphemism. You'll recognize that generation performs a larger feature than you ever imagined in this enterprise to lose yourself from tobacco. With each web page you switch, you cannot handiest get closer to being tobacco-free, but you may additionally turn out to be a professional at the workings of your personal mind. Would you need to emerge as the hold close of your neurological destiny?

Okay, take a deep breath and dive in, due to the reality what comes subsequent goes to plunge you into the deep layers of your being ready for the subsequent diploma of this journey? Here we skip.

Chapter 15: Neuroscience Of Tobacco

Have you ever felt as even though a few detail or a person else is controlling your movements, especially in phrases of smoking? Maybe it is time to look interior your brain, in which neural connections can also moreover offer some sudden solutions. Why is it vital to understand the neuroscience at the back of tobacco addiction? Simple: because it's within the mind in which the game is absolutely obtained or out of region.

Now right here's a few element to reflect onconsideration on. Imagine that your mind is an orchestra, a symphony of sports, impulses and reactions. Now suppose of every cigarette you slight as appearing like an underqualified conductor, disrupting the melody, difficult the musicians, and typically developing chaos. Would you need to hold to allow that underqualified conductor to take over?

This isn't always just hyperbole. Studies collectively with the best published in the mag Neuropharmacology (2015) have showed that nicotine can act as a brief-term cognitive enhancer, which can also initially make smoking seem beneficial. However, the rate is high: an preferred lower inside the thoughts's potential to feature optimally within the long term. In specific phrases, you may enjoy extra alert or targeted for a 2d, however ultimately, you're unbalancing the symphony that is your thoughts.

Imagine that you can input your mind as even though it have been a mansion with many rooms. Each room represents a selected mind feature: memory, interest, emotion and so forth. The cigarette, in this situation nicotine, acts like an insistent vacationer that starts offevolved offevolved last doorways, resetting alarms and cluttering rooms. Its have an effect on is insidious however effective. And now, could you actually need such an outsider to have manage over your precious domain?

You might also say, "But, wait! I'm gambling my life - what does it depend if I smoke?" The fact is, addiction isn't a sincere endeavor. It gives you small short-time period rewards even as quietly robbing you of your extended-time period freedom and functionality.

Have you ever taken into consideration why it feels so "particular" to smoke, no matter the truth that you apprehend it is wrong? It's due to the reality your brain has been programmed to are searching for rewards. But here's the capture: your mind can not tell the difference among a brief-term praise and a reward in order to advantage you ultimately. It's like a GPS that would simplest see the following flip in the street, but now not the very last excursion spot.

I can see you have got emerge as pensive, and rightly so. Because understanding how your thoughts have been hijacked by way of tobacco is the first step in reprogramming that complicated herbal laptop for your cranium. But don't worry, because of the reality there is a light on the cease of this tunnel, and it's miles no longer the glow of a lighter. It's the desire of liberated thoughts and liberated lifestyles.

You're getting ready to know-how how behavior is standard and maintained in that neural labyrinth that is your mind. So are you ready to dive into the neuroscience of techniques a cigarette, a few aspect so small and seemingly innocent, can hijack this form of complex and effective organ Because what follows will equip you with stronger and extra effective weapons in your fight to regain your freedom. And accept as true with me, you could want to be armed to the enamel for this struggle.

Ah, so what does this mind hijacking appear like from a neuroscientific mind-set? Before condemning your brain as a traitor for your purpose, it can pay to recognize what mechanisms are actually at play. Robert Sapolsky, a outstanding neurobiologist, unique in his e book "Behave: The Biology of Humans at Our Best and Worst" (2017) how neurotransmitters can basically hijack our reward and pride mechanisms. Nicotine, that key detail in cigarettes, is an professional at this shape of 'hijacking'.

So what takes place even as you inhale smoke from a cigarette? As nicotine enters your gadget, it is going right now on your mind and attaches to acetylcholine receptors, a neurotransmitter that plays a important role in cognitive function and reminiscence. This triggers a launch of numerous neurotransmitters, but the most brilliant is dopamine, the "revel in-particular" chemical. It is the equal neurotransmitter released inside the course of sports which includes consuming, having sex and achieving a purpose. Now agree with that whenever you smoke, you are sending a direct message to the reward middle of your mind that pronounces, "This is ideal. Do it all yet again."

You may be asking yourself, "If dopamine is proper, what is inaccurate with releasing it?". This is where things get complicated When you time and again flood your thoughts with dopamine artificially, like whilst you smoke, your mind adapts to the more with the useful resource of the use of reducing its very own natural dopamine production. This creates a vicious cycle. Smoking becomes the satisfactory way to sense "normal," due to the fact your thoughts now relies upon on outside stimuli to release dopamine.

The End of Food," a ebook thru Michael Pollan (2008), discusses how processed food creates a similar reaction in our brains. Like tobacco, positive meals are designed to be not possible to face up to, leading us to eat more than we need. It's the identical addiction mechanism, just with one-of-a-type materials. Your mind is a finite beneficial aid this is constantly being worn down with every impulsive preference you're making. The appropriate facts is that it is also pretty malleable and can be reprogrammed with the right stimuli.

Another crucial interest is how nicotine impacts the prefrontal cortex, the vicinity of the thoughts accountable for judgment and preference-making. Nicotine, as said neurologist Oliver Sacks factors out in "The Man Who Mistook His Wife for a Hat" (1985), no longer tremendous affects reminiscence and cognition, but additionally impacts your capability to make rational options. So, in a experience, it isn't always "you" who makes a desire to slight up that next cigarette, but a nicotine-altered brain.

I preference the ones elements have given you a cutting-edge-day mindset on how the act of smoking isn't always in truth a "dependancy" or a "preference," however the end result of an complex neurochemical orchestration designed to hold your dependancy. Don't fear, we are not doomed to be prisoners of our neurobiology. In truth, now which you recognise the enemy, you're in a better characteristic to counter their offensive. And be given as right with me, the following segment of this journey is designed to do genuinely that. Are you prepared to find out how you may reclaim authority over your non-public mind Because if you look at via, the fight on your freedom becomes more exciting and, extra importantly, extra practicable.

Okay, now that you have an information of methods tobacco and its additives like nicotine characteristic a form of chemical coup d'état on your mind, it is time to delve more deeply into the prolonged-term outcomes. Have you ever questioned what your mind might also additionally appear like in 10, 20, or 30 years if you maintain to smoke? Judith J. Prochaska, in "The Impact of Smoking on Mental Health" (2016), makes a disturbing argument about the risks of tobacco dependancy that pass beyond lung damage. We are talking about thoughts atrophy, quicker thoughts aging, and improved susceptibility to issues which includes despair and tension.

Let that idea take a seat for a 2d. Imagine that no longer handiest are you negative your lungs every time you mild up a cigarette, however you are accelerating the ageing of your brain. Visualize your mind as a sponge, absorbing every particle of nicotine and adapting, reworking itself to be more receptive to that brief and easy dose of dopamine. Think about how that, over the years, can also alternate the manner you are making decisions, the manner you method emotions, or even the way you have interplay with the people you care approximately. It's now not a quite image, is it?

Now, at this very 2nd, you have were given got the choice to exchange that route. Remember the idea of "neuroplasticity" that Norman Doidge mentioned in "The Brain That Changes Itself" (2007)? Your brain has the splendid functionality to reshape itself. Yes, the equal malleability that allowed tobacco dependancy to take root on your worrying gadget is what you can use in your benefit to banish it.

Want a tangible example? Let's have a observe the case of meditation. Researchers like Richard Davidson have shown that even a couple of minutes of every day meditation can trade the way our brains device feelings and react to strain. In his e-book "The Emotional Profile of Your Brain" (2012), Davidson delves into how meditation will let you take once more manage of your thoughts. Imagine the use of this sort of smooth and effective device to counteract the bad outcomes of nicotine on your mind. By converting your perception patterns, you may destroy the association among strain and smoking, accordingly weakening the chain of addiction.

But you may be asking yourself, "How do I get commenced out? Is it virtually feasible to change the form of my mind?" I even have an answer for you, and it's miles a effective certain. But you do not ought to take my word for it. In the following segment, we will dive deeper into powerful, era-based totally techniques in an effort to allow you to not only apprehend however reclaim your thoughts. Neuroscience is not virtually an proof of the manner you've got grow to be addicted; it is also the map a notable manner to manual you to freedom. Are you organized to embark on that adventure?

If you are right right here, when you have absorbed each word, each idea and each quote, it's far due to the fact you are already taking the first step inside the path of a fantastic lifestyles. Did you sense the transition? Every 2nd you spend money on information the neuroscience of smoking is one masses an awful lot much less minute given over to the poison of nicotine. But this isn't the surrender; it's miles without a doubt the top of a large iceberg that we want to find out collectively.

Let's recap for a 2nd. We started out this introspective journey by way of manner of addressing how tobacco launches a scientific attack in your thoughts's defenses, converting your chemistry for its very very own functions. We've visible that addiction isn't always a consider of lack of strength of will;

it's miles a depend of neurochemistry and mind shape. We've mentioned how neuroplasticity offers a doorway to restoration, a easy begin. We have touched on research and professionals inside the problem, which incorporates Judith J. Prochaska and Richard Davidson, who've supplied valuable statistics for understanding this thoughts maze.

Yes, we recognize that on every occasion you slight up a cigarette, you are reinforcing circuits on your mind that make you crave greater nicotine. But we moreover recognize that the mind can analyze and unlearn, trade and adapt. It's like an ever-flowing river; regardless of the reality that it is able to appear everyday, it is in a state of perennial exchange. And, if you look at the right strategies that we are capable of discover later, that river can be redirected.

Something notable awaits you within the subsequent chapter. You're going to discover about the "Butterfly Effect," a profound and transformative observe how small moves also can have a remarkable impact on your fight in the direction of tobacco addiction. Did you comprehend that a smooth exchange on your every day routine can be the cornerstone that in the long run crumbles the wall of dependancy? You do not want to miss out on that. So if you've got that cigarette to your hand right now, might not this be the ideal time to put it out and study on?

Let me depart you with this question: if you may regain control of your thoughts and, therefore, your life, what need to you be willing to do to acquire it? Keep it in mind as we drift forward, because in the following chapters, we are going to unfastened up the answers. You're approximately to discover that freedom isn't high-quality possible, however inevitable, if you observe the course we're charting collectively. Are you equipped to move beforehand? I knew it. See you in the subsequent financial disaster.

Chapter 16: The Butterfly Effect

Welcome to this new vicinity of readability and engagement. Have you ever at a loss for words how a clean flap of a butterfly's wings has to motive a storm at the possibility factor of the area? It sounds mystical, nearly a long way-fetched, however it's miles a metaphor deeply rooted in chaos concept that teaches us approximately how minute changes may additionally additionally have sizeable consequences. Imagine utilising this recognize-how to your journey to stop smoking. Yes, we're speakme about small changes-so small you'll barely have a look at them-however together they may wreck down the wall of addiction.

Don't allow your defend down; you're at a important point on your adventure. After exploring the neuroscience of smoking in Chapter 2, you may sense overwhelmed, even skeptical that this little "butterfly effect" want to work on something so ingrained in your mind. But what if you could control the variables to your everyday lifestyles so subtly which you would not even experience which encompass you had been growing a aware attempt to change?

Now, ask yourself: are you inclined to invest in the ones small changes to reap a large harvest of well being? It's about planting tiny seeds on the way to grow into sturdy flowers of resilience and strength of will. And if you expect this sounds too top notch to be genuine, think over again. In a enjoy, every preference you're making is like that flapping of a butterfly's wings.

Take a 2d to absorb this: have you ever ever ever taken into consideration that that cigarette you smoke within the direction of your espresso destroy might also absolutely be the precursor to a cycle of alternatives that lead to a whole day of smoking? It's as though one easy act devices in movement a sequence of activities with effects you can't even foresee. But if you may make one exchange, one so small which you barely take a look at it, have to you changed the path of your day?

It's not approximately breaking down partitions with a unmarried blow; it is about making small cracks within the edifice of addiction till the whole shape gives way and falls. The beauty of the Butterfly Effect lies in its simplicity and explosive potential.

Now, you will be asking yourself, "Okay, I recognize the idea, however how do I follow it in a realistic way?" Ah, expensive reader, that is in which the magic genuinely starts offevolved offevolved to take area. We're going to roll out a series of precise techniques, subsidized thru technological records, psychology and, certain, a piece precise juju magic as well, to convert your days and, ultimately, your life. Are you equipped to find out how a moderate flap of wings can unharness a hurricane of immoderate satisfactory exchange to your life?

If you are proper right here, it is because of the reality you've got got selected, consciously or unconsciously, to break some distance from the life you knew. You are equipped to unearth the hidden quantities of your psyche that have been acting as autopilots, guiding you toward the act of lights up again and again again. For a 2nd, allow bypass of your doubts. Are you prepared to take that first symbolic step, that preliminary flapping of wings?

The significance of the adjustments we communicate about right here need to not scare you. Think of them as levers. In his book "Think Big, Act Small" (2004), Jason Jennings talks approximately how small, consistent movements propel companies inside the route of prolonged-time period success. Now, what if we check that common experience to our crusade towards addiction? You can flip the ones small levers into your personal mechanism for engaging in huge effects.

Charles Duhigg, in his e-book "The Power of Habits" (2012), shows us that a addiction isn't always some thing extra than a clean equation: a signal, a ordinary and a praise.

The sign triggers the recurring that results in a reward. In your case, the signal is probably a second of strain, the recurring is lighting a cigarette, and the reward, oddly enough, is a short-term feel of treatment or delight. By converting actually one part of this equation, you could honestly dismantle a dangerous dependancy.

Duhigg's theories align perfectly with the Butterfly Effect concept. A diffused change in sign or ordinary can alternate the final consequences of the entire tool. Instead of accomplishing for that cigarette even as you experience stress, how approximately getting up and taking a short walk or having a tumbler of water? It may additionally seem insubstantial, however remember, small changes, huge outcomes.

Let's talk a hint about "substitutions". No, we do not propose taking a piece of sweet in place of a cigarette, no matter the fact that that can be useful for some. We endorse a deeper, greater intellectual substitution.

Viktor Frankl, in his big paintings "Man's Search for Meaning" (1946), talks approximately how one continuously has the liberty to choose out one's mind-set to any set of instances. So, while you feel the urge to smoke, can you pick out to look it as an possibility to work out your freedom to make a more wholesome preference?

Experts in chaos idea will say that the tool-your device of existence and alternatives-is continually in a country of flux, however interior that flux, there are patterns and structures that may be modified to alternate the entire gadget. The "weird attractors" are the ones elements in a chaotic machine that through hook or through manner of crook maintain it all together. In the existence of a smoker, that unusual attractor is probably the need for an "escape valve" in the form of a cigarette. Change the attractor and you exchange the entire tool.

You are approximately to discover how you may use this effective dynamic to turn the battle to stop smoking proper right into a adventure of self-discovery and boom. You'll dive into a sequence of examples, tips and techniques as a manner to take this idea from mere precept to each day practice. It's time to permit that wing flapping art work its magic. Are you organized for what's next?

Okay, you've got got immersed yourself in the idea; now how about experiencing its energy in exercise? Imagine you're in an aircraft, slowly trekking to an altitude in which ground troubles seem minuscule. At this altitude, your tobacco addiction seems small too, right? The reason for this extended mind-set is which you're about to get the complete image of the ripple consequences that tiny modifications can cause on your life. Now, will you allow me to walk you via an experience?

Remember the e-book "The 7 Habits of Highly Effective People" via way of Stephen Covey, posted in 1989. Covey proposes the concept of "beginning with an bring about thoughts." Here, permit's adapt that precept. Imagine a model of yourself that has completely kicked the smoking addiction. How do you revel in? How do you appearance? How do your clothes and home scent? Dive into the ones information.

Now, consider really one alternate you could make nowadays to move you inside the direction of that vision. It might be some aspect as easy as taking a particular course to art work to keep away from the store wherein you typically purchase cigarettes. Got it? Good.

In "Small Changes, Big Achievements" (2019), B.J. Fogg explains that the best adjustments are those that do not require an entire lot of motivation or strive, however that combine seamlessly into our each day exercise exercises. So that small exchange you genuinely identified, in case you do it proper, have to be some thing you could insert into your existence without an excessive amount of fuss.

Following up on the strength of workout, in "Willpower Is Not Enough" (1991), Arnold M. Washton and Donna Boundy argue that people regularly fail to surrender an addiction because of the fact they rely an excessive amount of on electricity of thoughts, ignoring outside elements that would make the adventure extra viable. For instance, if making a decision to take a detour to avoid the store in which you buy cigarettes, you're now not genuinely heading off a temptation; you're creating an surroundings that supports your intention.

But allow's make it greater tangible. Imagine that you normally spend 5 minutes a day shopping for cigarettes. If you select a course that avoids that save, the ones 5 minutes are freed up. What may also want to you do with that extra time? Maybe those 5 mins become the time you need to carry out a hint stretching wearing sports for you to make you revel in higher physical. Now, not best have you ever ever ever eliminated a horrible addiction, but you have got added a remarkable dependancy. And as all people understand, high-quality conduct tend to feed greater wonderful habits. Before you comprehend it, you may be gambling a series of latest wholesome behaviors, all brought on via one small change.

It's almost as if you've shifted your component of appeal, reorienting your entire device in the direction of a more wholesome pattern. This idea is harking back to Malcolm Gladwell's "The Tipping Point" (2000), which explores how small moves can bring about big modifications. Are you beginning to experience the functionality here? Can you be aware how this approach takes us out of the reductionism of "definitely quitting smoking" and right right right into a greater holistic technique to fitness?

this journey has involved you thus far, wait till you notice what comes subsequent. You've explored exchange from a microscopic attitude, now accept as true with the boom of those consequences for the duration of your lifestyles. As the butterfly impact in chaos concept indicates, a small change proper right here and now can result in incredible outcomes later. Doesn't it excite you to consider all the possibilities?

But it honestly isn't all. The next chapter will take you on a fascinating journey into your intestines. Yes, you study that right. You'll discover the mysterious and surprising courting amongst your intestine flowers and your dependancy to tobacco. Did you realise that what is going on on your gut want to have an effect on your thoughts and your choices? Intriguing, is not it?

So, armed with this new records and method, are you equipped to take the subsequent step for your journey to a tobacco-unfastened lifestyles? Because technological know-how, exercising and magic are approximately to return together in methods you in no way imagined. See you inside the subsequent financial smash.

Inhale deeply. Imagine that every breath you're taking takes you one step in the direction of the lifestyles you have got typically desired. Do you enjoy it? It's the enjoy of opportunity coursing through your veins, something you may in no manner enjoy via cigarette smoke.

In this exploration of the Butterfly Effect, you've got were given immersed yourself within the strength of small modifications. You've decided that a clean movement, which consist of resisting the urge to moderate up a cigarette, has the strength to alter the route of your life. The idea is as liberating as it's miles terrifying, but right right here you are, going through it. You've come to recognize that each small step counts and every conscious preference is a testomony on your developing self-control.

I need you to stop for a 2nd and remember all the authors stated and the concrete examples furnished. How do these theories and studies sense inside the workout of your lifestyles?

Edward Lorenz, the character in the back of the Butterfly Effect idea, in no manner imagined that his concept might be finished in such a lot of transformative approaches. Like Lorenz, your small act of resistance may also additionally want to have an impact past what you could accept as true with.

If you feel like this has already been an thrilling adventure, you want to recognise that we've got got slightly taken off. What you've got located out on this monetary disaster prepares you for what comes next; it's no longer anything brief of remarkable.

Imagine for a 2nd what it might be like if you can apprehend the connection between your brain and, nicely, your gut. Are you itching with hobby? You want to be. The next bankruptcy will take you into the enigma of your microbiota, the colony of microorganisms that stay to your gut, and its impact to your intellectual and physical health. Yes, even on your smoking behavior. If you have ever perplexed if there can be greater to tobacco dependancy than absolutely energy of will and mind chemistry, you will be satisfied to understand that there can be plenty more at play. And the most surprising detail is that the solution can be within the maximum unexpected region of all: your stomach.

With the clues we have were given had been given left at the roads we've got traveled and with the compass you presently preserve for your arms, I'll manual you thru discoveries that could flip the entirety you idea you knew approximately dependancy the wrong manner up. But, as always, the selection is yours. Are you prepared to take the following step on this adventure?

So, without further ado, permit's dive into the wonders of the unknown, of the surprising, of what is about to change your life all the time. See you within the subsequent monetary disaster.

Chapter 17: Controlling Addiction From The Micro Biota

Have you ever heard the announcing "You are what you eat"? While it is able to sound like a word off a present day day cereal field, the fact is that it's heaps deeper than you might imagine. Take a second to mirror on the complexity of your frame. From the folds and creases to your mind to the tiny capillaries that run via every inch of you, everything is intricately related.

Now, what if I cautioned you that interior you is an entire surroundings that plays a pivotal function on your fitness, mood and positive, even your capability to prevent smoking? Yes, you're approximately to embark on a journey at the manner to take you at once to the depths of your belly, wherein the microbiota - that community of microorganisms which are living on your gut - dictates a bargain more of your destiny than you may have ever imagined. Are you geared up to discover this surprising connection?

This financial disaster is essential due to the fact, as you come back to recognize how the microbiota affects your not unusual fitness, which consist of your smoking behavior, you may be capable of leverage that understanding to take manage of your lifestyles in a whole new and empowering way. Wouldn't or no longer it is extraordinary to recognize how a clean probiotic yogurt or nutritional choice ought to assist you prevent smoking? By the cease of this monetary break, that idea may not appear thus far-fetched.

If in Chapter 3 we pointed out the monumental impact that small changes ought to have on your lifestyles, thru the Butterfly Effect, here we are going to explore how some aspect as small as a bacteria in your gut can effect your mental and bodily well-being And if you're wondering how all of this connects to tobacco addiction, live with me. This is the start of a connection that could mark a earlier than and after in your path to quitting smoking.

The questions you may ask yourself as you discover this fascinating territory can range from "What is the real connection among my intestine and my thoughts?" to "Can I really control my impulses and desires thru my food plan?" Each answer will offer some different layer of data, now not simplest about how your frame works, but how you may make alternatives in case you need to advantage you in techniques you in no way imagined.

It's time to prevent thinking of you as a group of disconnected elements. Your frame and mind are one coherent entity, a extraordinary symbiosis of abilities that have an effect on each extraordinary in sudden methods. By information this connection, you could open the door to a worldwide of opportunities past any conventional approach of quitting smoking. So, luxurious reader, capture your imaginary magnifying glass and get prepared to get plenty, loads within the direction of your self. Are you prepared to get all the manner right down to the microscopic degree and find out how your gut can be the critical element to extinguishing that final cigarette?

Remember, the first step to trade is understanding, and you're approximately to advantage a big quantity of it. So maintain an open thoughts and keep with me on this interesting adventure. This is not virtually every different bankruptcy in your self-assist ebook; it's far a chapter in the e-book of your existence. And like numerous pinnacle ebook, each internet web page brings you towards the climax, the turning component you've got got been looking for Ready to show the internet internet web page?

Without a doubt, ultra-cutting-edge discoveries about the gut microbiota were cutting-edge. It is as although we've got discovered a current continent inner us, complete of opportunities and secrets to be uncovered. Emeran Mayer, in his ebook "The Mind-Gut Connection" (2016), defined in element how the trillions of microorganisms residing in our digestive tool aren't best essential for digestion, however moreover for our sizable intellectual fitness and properly-being.

In unique phrases, our gut is form of a second thoughts. Imagine for a second which you have a 2nd, extra primitive thoughts placed to your belly. Its language is tons less brand new, however its effect is further effective. Its strength can be in evaluation to that of the protagonist in a thriller acting inside the again of the curtains, silently maneuvering the threads of destiny. Does that sound sudden? It is. Reality often surpasses fiction.

If you've got ever questioned why positive factors make you feel a selected manner, or why your cravings appear to increase at the same time as you are forced, the answer might be there, in that intestine 'intelligence'. But how does all this have an effect for your smoking conduct? Could or not it's that the ones microorganisms are accomplices, or perhaps allies, on your combat in the path of nicotine?

Some research suggest that bacteria in our intestines can also additionally have an effect on how we metabolize materials, collectively with nicotine. For instance, a have a take a look at published inside the magazine Science in 2017 confirmed that notable bacteria of the genus Pseudomonas can smash down nicotine, thereby reducing its availability to the frame. In one of a kind phrases, the composition of your microbiota ought to even help you flush nicotine out of your tool faster. Now, anticipate for a second - may now not it's miles charming if a easy trade on your weight loss plan should adjust the bacterial composition of your gut, making it much less complicated with the intention to cease smoking?

If we've piqued your hobby, it is because we are gambling chords to a song that has generally been there, but to which you could now not have paid sufficient interest. In "The Hidden Half of Nature" (2016), authors David R. Bernard Law 1st viscount montgomery of alamein and Anne Biklé delve into the arena of the microbiome, explaining how these microorganisms have an effect on everything from our intellectual health to our capability to combat illness. Could or not it's that moreover they play a characteristic in addiction? Evidence suggests they do.

And in case you're questioning that probably you've got already were given too many things to worry approximately for your quit smoking journey, save you for a 2d. Instead of seeing this as another burden, what if we determined it as each other tool on your quitting toolbox? In Chapter 2, we immersed you inside the neuroscience of smoking to expose you strategies your thoughts has been hijacked with the aid of the use of the usage of cigarettes. Now, believe that this data approximately your microbiota gives you a shape of "administrator password" to regain manage.

So, what are you going to do with this statistics that has fallen to you need a treasure chest inside the center of the ocean?

Are you going to open it to discover its riches or allow it sink into the depths of "I'll attempt all over again later"? The choice is to your hands, or probably I ought to say, on your stomach.

Let's maintain navigating this ocean whole of surprises, opportunities and positive, worrying conditions. Are you prepared for the following discovery? Do you experience geared up to add a powerful new resource in your give up smoking arsenal? Keep your hobby alive; it's miles your compass on this interesting adventure. And believe me, the following bankruptcy has even more treasures to provide, especially in the area of rebooting your tastes. Are you prepared to rediscover the flavors that dependancy stole from you? Ah, however it truely is a story for yet again. Now, allow's maintain delving into the fascinating worldwide of the microbiota. Ready to dive even deeper?

So, there we are, right sailing together in this adventure to freedom, with a treasure trove of expertise in our fingers. Now, allow's delve into sensible examples. In some strategies, concept without software program is sort of a recipe we in no way cook dinner dinner: it seems best on paper, but it never nourishes us.

Let me percent a tale that illustrates how microbiota can play a critical role in our behavior. David Perlmutter, in his ebook "Brain Maker: The Power of Gut Microbes to Heal and Protect Your Brain-for Life" (2015), relates the case of a lady who suffered from anxiety and excessive temper swings. When she adjusted her diet regime to nurture a more in shape microbiome, her signs and symptoms advanced dramatically. Now, I'm no longer telling you that converting your microbiota will treatment all of your problems. But what if I recommended you that it may be a key factor in the quitting equation?

www.ingramcontent.com/pod-product-compliance
Lightning Source LLC
Chambersburg PA
CBHW071446080526
44587CB00014B/2009